fat BURNING FOODS COOKBOOK

Edited by Betty Bianconi, R.D.

Ottenheimer
PUBLISHERS

Created and manufactured by Ottenheimer Publishers, Inc.
© 1995 Ottenheimer Publishers, Inc.
10 Church Lane, Baltimore, Maryland 21208, USA
All rights reserved
Printed in the United States of America
CB-731A

CONTENTS

INTRODUCTION

by Judy Jameson, author of
Fat-Burning Foods and Other Weight-Loss Secrets

THANK YOU, READERS. AND CONGRATULATIONS!

Your support and enthusiasm have turned our book, *Fat-Burning Foods and Other Weight-Loss Secrets,* into a runaway best-seller. Hundreds and thousands of people have now learned that you can be more slender and more energetic than ever before, without hunger.

The amazing discoveries revealed in *Fat-Burning Foods and Other Weight-Loss Secrets* have taught readers that you do not have to travel the road to a slender new you on an empty stomach. **You do not have to be hungry to lose weight!**

Many of you have discovered that the recipes in *Fat-Burning Foods and Other Weight-Loss Secrets* were delicious as well as satisfying. But there was a problem—there weren't enough of them! So here's an entire book of recipes that will help you keep incorporating "fat-burning foods" into your meals. This book is our way of helping you keep your commitment to good health.

Before you begin browsing through these mouth-watering recipes, let's review your program for permanent weight loss.

Why Dieting Doesn't Work

"Fad-of-the-month" dieting causes more harm than good, because every time you starve yourself, your body's survival instinct kicks in and actively tries to preserve its fat stores. And your body becomes more efficient at hanging on to its fat with every successive diet. So when you go off one of these diets—and just about everyone does, because your body eventually wants to start eating normally again—not only do you gain all the weight back, but you likely end up heavier than ever. This is the vicious cycle many dieters know so well: lose 10 pounds, gain back 15, lose those 15 pounds, then gain back 20, and so on.

Eventually, conventional dieting will slow your metabolism down so much that even small portions of food can make you gain weight. **Starvation diets are the problem—not the solution—for overweight people.**

One of the keys to success in this exciting program is that you are never hungry. Your body never thinks it's starving, so you can keep burning off that fat, slowly and steadily.

To get off the "yo-yo-diet" syndrome of weight loss followed by weight gain, you must eat enough food to keep your metabolic rate up. **Your diet must contain at least 10 calories per pound of your ideal body weight.** In other words, if you want to weigh 120 pounds, you should be eating at least 1,200 calories every day.

The best way for you to lose weight permanently is to:

➤ eat the fat-burning foods on this program, and

➤ raise your metabolic rate through moderate exercise.

Miracle Foods Every Day Keep the Waistline at Bay

"Miracle" foods high in complex carbohydrates are the foundation of the *Fat-Burning Foods* program. These foods, which include fruits, vegetables, legumes, brans, grains, cereals, pasta, rice, potatoes and bread, not only are extremely nutritious, satisfying and inexpensive, but also are extraordinary fat-burning tools.

Here is the list of the 30 amazing fat-burning foods as it originally appeared in *Fat-Burning Foods and Other Weight-Loss Secrets*. These foods are all high in complex carbohydrates and low in fat. They are also the foundation of most of the recipes in this book. Whenever you feel the urge, grab (or cook) one of these miracle foods and eat until you're satisfied.

30 Fat-Burning Foods

Apples
Bananas
Beans (all varieties)
Bread (plain)
Broccoflower
Broccoli
Cabbage
Cauliflower
Celery
Citrus fruit
Corn, including
    air-popped popcorn
Cranberries
Grains and grain products
Grapes
Jam (sugar-free,
    low-cal only)
Leeks
Lettuce
Melons
Mushrooms
Pasta (low-fat,
    preferably whole-grain)
Pears
Peas
Peppers
Pineapple
Potatoes
Root vegetables
Spinach
Tomatoes
Waffles and pancakes
    (frozen, low-fat)
Zucchini

Why Does This Program Take Off Pounds?

Scientists aren't sure why, but your body seems to handle complex carbohydrates differently than it does other types of food. Meals high in complex carbohydrates appear to raise the metabolic rates of overweight people more than meals containing a comparable number of calories made up mostly of fats or proteins. Furthermore, your body seems to "prefer" complex carbohydrates to fats for energy. A number of studies now indicate that it's "easier" for the body to convert carbohydrates into energy and dietary fat into body fat for future use. Perhaps dietary fat is so similar in chemical composition to our body fat that it just takes less energy to convert it into flab. These foods seem to lose many of their calories just in the process of digestion! **Calories from starch, sugar and other carbohydrates are not stored in your body as easily as calories from fat.**

Although you don't need to count calories on this program, the truth is that complex carbohydrates don't have a lot of calories. Not only will foods rich in complex carbohydrates provide the same energy ounce for ounce as protein, but they have less than half the calories of fat. You can eat as much as you want of these foods to satisfy your appetite. In fact, your appetite is "cued" to tell your body to stop eating during the time your body converts energy from carbohydrates into glucose for energy.

Fortunately, complex carbohydrates are also very good for you. Because they break down easily into glucose (blood sugar), your main source of energy, these foods are like high-octane, clean-burning fuel for your body. Not incidentally, they're also high in dietary fiber and may well reduce your risk of diseases such as cancer. **Your body prefers to fuel itself with carbohydrate calories.**

The two main types of dietary fiber, water-soluble and insoluble fiber, are both excellent for weight control and for your health.

Water-soluble fiber is a type of fiber that can dissolve in water. It's found in foods such as oat bran and in many legumes, fruits and vegetables. In general, these foods help regulate blood sugar levels and may also lower cholesterol levels in your blood. The soluble fiber in apples and oats has also been linked to reduced risk of heart disease.

Insoluble fiber, found in foods like wheat bran, peanuts and many legumes, fruits and vegetables, provides bulk to keep your digestive system in good order. It is the roughage your digestive system needs to stay healthy, acting like a toothbrush on the interior of your digestive tract. It therefore reduces your risk of constipation, hemorrhoids, diverticular disease and possibly some cancers. The insoluble fiber in wheat bran has been linked with reduced risk of colon cancer and possibly breast cancer.

Like other complex carbohydrate foods, fiber helps satisfy hunger and thus helps you resist the temptation to overload on fat. Fiber in your diet adds necessary bulk and is satisfying. It takes a long time to chew most fibrous foods, which gives time for the "I'm full" signal to reach your brain.

All of which leads to two simple conclusions:

➤ The bulk of your diet should come from complex carbohydrates.

➤ Plan to eat 30 to 40 grams of fiber every day.

Fats: Just Say No

Fats, found in most meats, dairy products, nuts and grain products, are necessary for your health. But the average North American diet comprises a hugely excessive 35% to 40% fat, thanks to our fondness for red meat, fried foods, dairy products and desserts. And all you really need to satisfy your body's minimum requirements is the equivalent of a daily teaspoon of canola oil. You'll get at least that if you eat the minimum protein recommendations of this program.

The problem with too much fat in your diet is that calories from fat are more likely to "stick to your waistline" than calories from carbohydrates and protein. Fat calories are also harder to burn off than carbohydrates and protein. And they're more readily converted to body fat, since your body prefers to use carbohydrate calories for fuel. The more fat you eat, the more likely you are to be overweight—and stay overweight. **Fat consumption is the critical factor in obesity.** You must reduce your fat intake to 20% to 30% of your daily calories, preferably less.

Cutting down your fat intake is also essential for your good health. Studies show that a low-fat diet can make fatty deposits in coronary arteries start to shrink, especially if you also quit smoking, exercise sensibly and keep the stress in your life under control.

All fats are bad for your waistline. Saturated fats (the kind found in red meat and butter) are the most obvious source of fat in your diet. You must cut down your intake of red meat to a maximum of 5 ounces per serving, no more than twice a week. The rest of your meat intake should consist of chicken and fish.

The fat in dairy products is another fat-maker on you. You must switch to skim milk and low-fat cheese products and limit your daily consumption of them to a maximum of 2 cups of skim milk or the equivalent amount of low-fat yogurt or cottage cheese. Avoid butter, whole milk and hard cheese.

Oils, margarine and other "pure" fats, such as those found in most commercial salad dressings, should be avoided as much as possible. And although vegetables are one of the mainstays of this program, some vegetables, such as avocados and olives, are loaded with fat and should also be avoided. **Eat as little fat as possible, from all sources.**

Protein: Too Much, Too Often

You need a new supply of protein every day to repair and build almost all body tissues and to produce virtually every chemical in your body.

The trouble is, most people consume too much meat and cheese and not enough potatoes and bread. A person whose daily intake is 2,000 calories requires only 200 to 400 calories of protein from animals a day, which you can get from 6 ounces of broiled fish and an ounce or two of cottage cheese. Another way of calculating this is to realize that you need only about an ounce of protein for every 18 pounds of ideal body weight. In other words, a 126-pound woman needs only about 7 ounces of protein, and a 162-pound man needs about 9 ounces of protein in a day.

You can easily reduce your overall protein intake by filling up on healthy fat-burning complex carbohydrates instead.

Skim milk, low-fat yogurt, and low-fat cheeses are a good source of calcium and protein and can be consumed in limited quantities. You can also eat small amounts of eggs, beef, pork and chicken and still lose weight.

Plan to eat one or two dinners of lean red meat weekly, one or two dinners featuring chicken, one or two of fish, and *at least* one vegetarian dinner a week. Never eat more than 5 ounces of protein from animal sources in a day. **You need only a maximum of 10% to 15% of your daily calories from protein.**

Exercising: Get a Move On!

Your basal metabolic rate, the speed at which your body burns off calories, is an important factor in your ability to lose weight and keep it off. Food alone won't do the trick. Only regular activity will keep your metabolism high enough to keep the fat-burning action going. Simple, moderate exercise on a regular basis will keep your metabolism high enough to ensure maximum fat burning. Hours after activity, your basal metabolic rate remains raised. **Regular activity will keep your metabolism high enough to keep that body fat burning off.**

Not insignificantly, exercise also makes you feel more energetic and good about yourself. You'll sleep better, cope with stress better, deal with the ups and downs of life more calmly. That feeling of vitality can only help you—and your eating program—in the long run.

What type of exercise is best for weight loss? Believe it or not, you don't have to "go for the burn" to maximize fat-burning potential. In fact, if you work too hard at your workout, your body could stop drawing on your fat stores for food and start depending on your carbohydrate supplies.

Especially if you're older than 45, you should avoid high-impact aerobic activities, like jogging and jumping, which force too much sudden weight onto joints and the lower back. And you must certainly take competitive sports with a grain of salt. They're too hard on your system and not necessary for weight loss. Your victory will be a new slim body, not first prize at the Boston Marathon.

An activity like walking is absolutely the best form of exercise. Find a half-hour a few times a week, mark it down on your calendar and set aside that time in your schedule for the next few months. Your waistline will reap the benefits.

Summing Up: the Basic Rules for This Amazing Weight-loss Program

➤ Eat as much as you want of the 30 fat-burning foods.

➤ Enjoy as many complex carbohydrate foods as you need to feel full, such as fruits, vegetables and grains. These foods must provide at least 65% of your daily calories.

➤ Aim to eat at least 30 to 40 grams of fiber daily. To keep your fiber intake up, read package labels and always buy the higher-fiber product (it's usually lower in fat, too!).

➤ Consume no more than 20% to 30% of your total daily calories as fat. To keep life simple, avoid fat when possible.

➤ Up to 10% to 15% of your daily calories can come from animal sources of protein.

➤ Eat no more than 5 ounces of animal protein in a day and no more than two dinners of lean red meat a week.

➤ Eat at least one vegetarian dinner a week—preferably two.

➤ Eat as little hard cheese as possible and even low-fat varieties in moderation.

➤ Drink up to 2 cups of skim milk a day, or eat the equivalent amount of low-fat yogurt or cottage cheese.

➤ Enjoy regular activity such as a brisk daily walk; it will keep your metabolism high enough to burn that body fat off.

A Word of Warning

Following this program will improve your health, but before making changes to your diet or activity level, discuss your decision with your physician. This book is designed to enhance your physician's prescribed treatment, not replace it.

Using This Book from Morning to Night

Let's take a quick look at how you can use this book, starting with breakfast.

A good breakfast is essential for weight loss. One Midwestern study showed that overweight people who received their entire allotment of the day's calories at breakfast lost weight, whereas those who took in all their calories at dinnertime gained weight. You wouldn't jump in your car and go on a big trip without filling your gas tank! So why would you even consider starting your day without a good breakfast?

Break away from the expected and eat leftovers from last night's dinner for breakfast. The Garbanzo Bean Salad (page 55), Broccoli Casserole (page 84), Noodles Milanese (page 118), and even Lentil Soup (page 36) in this book are just as nutritious in the morning as they were the night before.

As the day progresses, some of the same people who skip breakfast also think that a quick lunch on the go will help them lose weight. They're wrong. Lunches on the go tend to be long on fat and short on satisfaction. Plan a fat-burning meal that you can relax and enjoy if only for 20 minutes.

Consider fresh fruit, a sandwich of low-fat cheese, turkey or chicken breast, a fillet of fish, with lettuce and tomato, sliced vegetables or leftovers warmed up from dinner. Spice up your sandwiches with low-fat mayonnaise, ketchup, salsa or mustard rather than butter or margarine. If you're in a rush, consider beans on toast or cold rice salad.

If you're a soup fan, the soup recipes (pages 20 to 38) will really provide you with midday satisfaction. A big bowl of chowder will fill you up and keep you going. Dry soup to which you add water is also a good low-fat bet. Whatever soup you choose, stick to clear broths rather than cream soups.

Toward sunset, the temptation to overeat could feel overwhelming. You're relaxed, maybe a little tired after the challenges of your day, and stuffing yourself into oblivion looks like a pretty appealing prospect. Stop!

You can accompany the entrées in this book with relatively large portions of baked potatoes, whole grains, vegetables, salads splashed with low-fat dressing, and fruits. Consult the salad and side dish sections for inspiration. And eat dinner no later than 5 to 6 P.M. to give your body time to digest the meal before bedtime.

Fat-Burning Flavor Boosters

The nutritional information accompanying each recipe in this book is based on its basic ingredients. But don't forget that garnishes or other additions could add fat or calories. You can, however, use the following condiments and sauces to zip up your food:

Bouillon cubes	Mint sauce
Chili sauce	Mustards
Clear broth	Pickles
Cocktail sauce	Relishes
Cranberry sauce	Salsa
Herbs	Soy sauce
Horseradish	Spices
Ketchup	Steak sauce
Lemon juice	Sweet-and-sour sauces
Lime juice	Vinegars
Low-fat mayonnaise	Worcestershire sauce

Keep in mind that many of these condiments, while low in fat, are high in sodium. Many are available in reduced sodium and lower fat varieties.

Conclusion

As you've already learned, this program is incredibly easy to follow. It involves no calorie counting, no complicated calculations, no specialized foods or food combinations—and no more hunger pangs.

So here is an array of exciting new experiments in eating. These recipes will take you from breakfast to bedtime and to a new, slim, health-conscious you.

HOW TO READ THE
NUTRITION INFORMATION

The *Fat-Burning Foods Cookbook* includes another helpful tool to assist you with your meal planning. Each recipe features nutrition information, which includes:

Calories	Consume at least 10 calories per pound of your ideal body weight.
Protein	Only 10% to 15% of your daily calories should come from animal sources of protein. To determine the percentage of calories from protein, multiply the grams of protein by 4, divide that number by the number of calories, and multiply by 100.
Fat	Consume no more than 65 grams a day.
% fat calories	No more than 20% to 30% of your daily calories should come from fat. Remember, it's your total consumption over the whole day that's important, not the percentage in one food or meal.
Cholesterol	Consume no more than 300 mg. daily.
Carbohydrates	These are good for you! At least 65% of your daily calories should come from complex carbohydrates. To determine the percentage of calories from carbohydrates, multiply the grams of carbohydrates by 4, divide that number by the number of calories, and multiply by 100.
Sodium	Keep this under 2,400 mg. daily.
Fiber	Eat 30 to 40 grams every day.

SEVEN-DAY MENU

Day 1

Breakfast   1 cup tomato juice
             1 orange
             1 low-fat frozen waffle
             1 Whole-Wheat Date Biscuit (page 68)

Lunch   Green and Yellow Pasta (page 99)
             1 sliced tomato
             Ginger Muffin (page 65)

Dinner   Curried Chicken Salad (page 42)
             Nutty Brown Bread (page 75)
             Cranberry Ice (page 165)

Snack   1 banana

Day 2

Breakfast   1 cup orange juice
            1 slice cantaloupe melon
            1 ounce prepared cereal with ¼ cup skim milk
            1 Oatmeal Muffin (page 63)

Lunch   1 Lentil Burger on a whole-wheat pita
               (page 104)
            Cucumbers in Dill (page 130)
            1 apple

Dinner   Gazpacho (page 26)
            Mediterranean Baked Fish (page 124)
            Marinated Vegetables (page 131)
            1 slice Peachy Yogurt Pie (page 181)

Snack   1 cup air-popped popcorn

Day 3

Breakfast   1 cup apple juice
½ grapefruit
½ cup cooked oatmeal with cinnamon
and raisins
1 slice Banana Bread (page 78)

Lunch   Health Salad (page 46)
1 slice Nutty Brown Bread (page 75)
1 orange

Dinner   Beef and Bean Soup (page 28)
Corn Bread (page 73)
Small mixed greens salad with fat-free dressing
1 slice Upside-Down Cake (page 172)

Snack   ½ cup grapes

Day 4

Breakfast   1 cup orange juice
             1 apple
             1 ounce prepared cereal with ¼ cup skim milk
             1 Applesauce Banana Muffin (page 66)

Lunch   Curried Chicken Salad (page 42)
             ½ cup steamed broccoli
             ½ cup applesauce

Dinner   Stuffed Squash (page 89)
             Spanish Rice (page 143)
             Whole-Wheat Irish Soda Bread (page 77)
             Frozen Pineapple Yogurt (page 184)

Snack   1 slice Banana Bread (page 78)

Day 5

Breakfast   1 cup pineapple juice
½ cup hot cereal topped with fresh blueberries
1 Ginger Muffin (page 65)

Lunch   Beef and Bean Soup (page 28)
1 slice Nutty Brown Bread (page 75)
Frozen Pineapple Yogurt (page 184)

Dinner   Sole with Sweet-Sour Vegetables (page 122)
Orange Rice (page 141)
Honey Corn Muffin (page 61)
Fresh Harvest Pie (page 174)

Snack   1 apple

Day 6

Breakfast   1 cup orange juice
            1 low-fat frozen pancake topped with fresh
                strawberries
            1 Whole-Wheat Date Biscuit (page 68)

Lunch   Tomatoes Stuffed with Chicken (page 109)
            Corn Bread (page 73)
            1 Carrot-Date Bar (page 177)

Dinner   Eggplant Italiano (page 86)
            Spinach Salad Veronique (page 47)
            Ambrosia (page 171)

Snack   1 cup carrot sticks

Day 7

Breakfast   1 cup tomato juice
1 slice honeydew melon
1 ounce prepared cereal with ¼ cup skim milk,
    topped with sliced bananas

Lunch   1 All Green and White Sandwich (page 100)
Oven French Fries (page 148)
Frozen Pineapple Yogurt (page 184)

Dinner   Sweet-and-Sour Cabbage Soup (page 31)
Moo Goo Gai Pan (page 111)
Steamed Brown Bread (page 71)
Orange Sherbet (page 182)

Snack   1 pear

SAVORY SOUPS

Green Pepper Soup

3   tablespoons butter
½   cup chopped green peppers
½   cup chopped onions
2   cups defatted chicken broth or bouillon
¼   teaspoon dried oregano
2   tablespoons flour
¼   teaspoon salt
1   cup skim milk
     Chopped green peppers for garnish

Melt 1 tablespoon butter in large saucepot over medium heat. Sauté peppers and onions until onions are golden. Add chicken broth or bouillon and oregano. Reduce heat to low; simmer for 10 minutes. Place in blender; carefully puree for a few seconds.

In same saucepot, melt remaining 2 tablespoons butter; stir in flour and salt. Cook, stirring, until bubbly. Remove from heat. Gradually stir in milk. Return to heat; cook, stirring, until thickened and smooth. Stir in blended green pepper mixture. Serve hot or cold, sprinkled with chopped green peppers. Makes 4 servings.

Per serving: 141 calories; 5 g. protein; 9 g. fat; 61% calories from fat; 24 mg. cholesterol; 8 g. carbohydrates; 626 mg. sodium; trace g. fiber

Puree of Vegetable Soup

2   medium onions, sliced
2   tablespoons butter or margarine
4   cups water
1½   pounds beef with bones for soup
3   ribs celery, cut into large pieces
3   medium carrots, cut into large pieces
2   medium potatoes, peeled and cut into large pieces
1   large parsnip, peeled and cut into large pieces
5   sprigs fresh parsley
1½   teaspoons salt
¼   teaspoon ground white pepper
1   tablespoon snipped fresh dill, or 1 teaspoon dried
     dill

Melt butter or margarine in large saucepot over medium heat. Sauté onions until golden. Add water, bones, celery, carrots, potatoes, parsnip, parsley, salt and pepper. Bring to boil. Reduce heat to low; cover and simmer for 2 hours or until meat is tender.

Remove meat and bones from broth; reserve for future use. With slotted spoon, remove vegetables and transfer to food processor, blender or food mill. Puree until smooth; return mixture to broth with dill. Heat through. Makes 8 servings.

Per serving: 72 calories; 1 g. protein; 1 g. fat; 19% calories from fat; 3 mg. cholesterol; 13 g. carbohydrates; 442 mg. sodium; 2 g. fiber

Quick Tuna Chowder

1   can (7 ounces) solid white tuna packed in oil
1   large onion, chopped
3   cups water
2   large potatoes, peeled and thinly sliced
½   teaspoon salt
¼   teaspoon pepper
¼   teaspoon dried oregano
1   can (10¾ ounces) condensed tomato soup
1   tablespoon chopped fresh parsley (optional)

Drain oil from tuna; measure 2 tablespoons reserved oil into large heavy saucepan. Flake and reserve tuna. Add onions to oil in saucepan; cook over low heat, stirring often, until soft. Stir in water, potatoes, salt, pepper and oregano. Cover and cook 15 minutes, or just until potatoes are tender. Stir in undiluted tomato soup and flaked tuna. Simmer 5 minutes to blend flavors. Sprinkle with parsley, if desired. Makes 4 servings.

Per serving: 278 calories; 18 g. protein; 8 g. fat; 27% calories from fat; 28 mg. cholesterol; 33 g. carbohydrates; 979 mg. sodium; 2 g. fiber

Vegetable-Burger Soup

½ pound lean ground beef
2 cups water
1 can (16 ounces) stewed tomatoes
1 can (8 ounces) tomato sauce
1 package (10 ounces) frozen mixed vegetables
½ envelope (¼ cup) dry onion soup mix
1 teaspoon sugar

In large heavy saucepan over medium heat, lightly brown ground beef; drain off fat. Stir in remaining ingredients. Bring to boil. Reduce heat; cover and simmer for 20 minutes. Makes 8 servings.

Per serving: 120 calories; 9 g. protein; 5 g. fat; 40% calories from fat; 24 mg. cholesterol; 9 g. carbohydrates; 337 mg. sodium; 2 g. fiber

Minestrone

4   ounces dried white beans, rinsed and picked over
9¼ cups water
2   medium onions, sliced
2   cloves garlic, minced
1   slice bacon, chopped
2   tablespoons olive oil
2   large tomatoes, chopped
½   cup red wine
1   tablespoon fresh oregano, or 1 teaspoon dried oregano
2   medium carrots, peeled and diced
2   ribs celery, diced
2   small potatoes, peeled and diced
1   small turnip, peeled and diced
½   small cabbage (about 8 ounces), shredded
½   cup uncooked macaroni or other small pasta
    Salt and pepper to taste
    Grated Parmesan cheese (optional)

In large saucepot or Dutch oven, place beans in 1¼ cups water; let stand overnight.

In large skillet over medium heat, sauté onions, garlic and bacon in oil until bacon is cooked. Add tomatoes, wine and oregano. Boil rapidly 5 minutes, or until liquid is reduced. Add bacon mixture to beans; stir in remaining 8 cups water. Bring to boil. Reduce heat to low; cover and simmer 1½ hours.

Add carrots, celery, potatoes and turnip. Cover and simmer 30 minutes. Add cabbage and macaroni. Cover and simmer 15 minutes more, until macaroni is tender. Season with salt and pepper. Top with cheese, if desired. Makes 6 servings.

Per serving: 266 calories; 8 g. protein; 8 g. fat; 28% calories from fat; 0 mg. cholesterol; 39 g. carbohydrates; 89 mg. sodium; 8 g. fiber

Beet Soup

 1 can (16 ounces) whole beets
2½ cups water
 1 small onion, finely chopped, or ½ teaspoon onion salt
 1 teaspoon sour or regular salt
 1 teaspoon sugar
    Nonfat sour cream (optional)

Drain beets, reserving liquid, and shred coarsely.

In medium saucepan, place beets, reserved liquid, water, onions or onion salt, salt and sugar. Bring to boil. Top with sour cream, if desired. Makes 4 servings.

Per serving: 44 calories; 1 g. protein; 0 g. fat; 3% calories from fat; 0 mg. cholesterol; 10 g. carbohydrates; 832 mg. sodium; 2 g. fiber

Gazpacho

2   cups tomato juice
1   cup finely chopped peeled tomatoes
½   cup finely chopped green peppers
½   cup finely chopped celery
½   cup finely chopped cucumbers
¼   cup minced onions
1   clove garlic, minced
2   tablespoons tarragon vinegar
2   tablespoons olive oil
2   teaspoons chopped fresh parsley
1   teaspoon chopped fresh, frozen or freeze-dried chives
1   teaspoon salt
½   teaspoon Worcestershire sauce
¼   teaspoon pepper

In large bowl or container, stir all ingredients until well blended. Cover tightly; chill at least 4 hours. Stir just before serving. Makes 6 servings.

Per serving: 66 calories; 1 g. protein; 4 g. fat; 59% calories from fat; 0 mg. cholesterol; 6 g. carbohydrates; 667 mg. sodium; 1 g. fiber

Chili Bean Soup

1   package (16 ounces) pink, red or pinto beans,
      rinsed and picked over
7   cups water
1   teaspoon garlic salt
1   teaspoon onion salt
¼   teaspoon dried thyme
¼   teaspoon dried marjoram
1   can (10½ ounces) condensed beef or chicken broth
1   can (16 ounces) stewed tomatoes
1   package (1⅜ ounces) chili seasoning mix or 1 can
      (7 ounces) green chili salsa

In large saucepot or Dutch oven, place beans and enough water to cover; let stand overnight.

Add 6 cups water, garlic salt, onion salt, thyme and marjoram. Bring to boil. Reduce heat to low; cover and simmer 2½ to 3 hours, or until beans are tender. Add hot water as needed to keep moist.

Remove 3 cups cooked beans; save for another use. With potato masher or fork, mash remaining beans with their liquid. Add remaining ingredients and 1 cup hot water. Cook 10 minutes, or until heated through. Makes 6 servings.

Per serving: 126 calories; 7 g. protein; 0 g. fat; 6% calories from fat; 0 mg. cholesterol; 23 g. carbohydrates; 476 mg. sodium; 10 g. fiber

Beef and Bean Soup

1½ packages (16 ounces each) dried beans of any combination (lentils, lima, navy, pinto, black turtle, black-eyed peas, red kidney), rinsed and picked over
1 pound beef bones with meat for soup
4½ quarts water
2 cloves garlic, minced
1 tablespoon dried basil, or to taste
2 teaspoons dried thyme, or to taste
2 teaspoons lemon pepper, or to taste
3 large potatoes, cut into bite-size pieces
1 can (28 ounces) crushed tomatoes
Salt to taste

In large saucepot or Dutch oven, place beans in enough water to cover; let stand overnight.

If desired, brown bones in large skillet over medium heat. Add bones to undrained beans. Stir in water, garlic, basil, thyme and lemon pepper. Bring to boil. Reduce heat to low; cover and simmer 1½ hours, or until beans are just tender.

Stir in potatoes and tomatoes. Cook 15 to 25 minutes more, or until potatoes and beans are fully tender. Remove bones. Season with salt. Makes 24 servings.

Per serving: 116 calories; 7 g. protein; 1 g. fat; 8% calories from fat; 5 mg. cholesterol; 20 g. carbohydrates; 61 mg. sodium; 6 g. fiber

Mushrooms in Broth

1½ cups sliced dried mushrooms
2   cups chicken broth or stock
1   green onion
1   slice (½ inch) fresh ginger
¼   cup soy sauce
1   tablespoon cornstarch, mixed with 2 tablespoons
    cold water
1   teaspoon sugar
1   teaspoon salt

In medium saucepan, place mushrooms and broth or stock; let stand 30 minutes.

Add onion and ginger. Bring just to boil. Reduce heat to low; cover and simmer 1 hour. Remove and discard onion and ginger. Stir in remaining ingredients. Cook over medium heat, stirring constantly, until smooth and slightly thickened. Makes 5 servings.

Per serving: 100 calories; 5 g. protein; 0 g. fat; 6% calories from fat; 0 mg. cholesterol; 21 g. carbohydrates; 1563 mg. sodium; 7 g. fiber

Meat and Vegetable Soup

8   cups water
1½   pounds beef bones with meat for soup
1   can (16 ounces) tomatoes
2   ribs celery, chopped
1   medium onion, chopped
½   medium green pepper, seeded and chopped
½   cup dry lima beans
3   tablespoons large pearl barley
½   small bunch parsley, chopped
2   medium carrots, peeled and diced
1   medium sweet potato, peeled and cubed
1   can (16 ounces) drained green beans, or 1 package
         (10 ounces) frozen green beans
1   can (16 ounces) drained peas, or 1 package
         (10 ounces) frozen peas
1   can (8 ounces) creamed-style corn
1   can (8 ounces) tomato sauce
      Salt and pepper to taste

In large saucepot or Dutch oven, place 4 cups water, bones, undrained tomatoes, celery, onions, green peppers, lima beans, barley and parsley. Bring to boil. Reduce heat to medium-low; cover and cook 2 hours.

Add remaining ingredients and remaining 4 cups water. Cook 45 to 55 minutes more, or until vegetables and meat are tender. Remove bones. Season with salt and pepper. Makes 12 servings.

Per serving: 157 calories; 10 g. protein; 3 g. fat; 19% calories from fat; 20 mg. cholesterol; 22 g. carbohydrates; 285 mg. sodium; 6 g. fiber

Sweet-and-Sour Cabbage Soup

8   cups water
2   pounds short ribs or beef chuck, fat removed
1   large onion, sliced
1   head (about 2 pounds) cabbage, shredded
2   cans (16 ounces) stewed tomatoes
½   cup sugar
3   tablespoons lemon juice
1   teaspoon salt
½   teaspoon ground ginger
¼   teaspoon pepper

In large saucepot over high heat, place water, chuck or short ribs and onions. Bring to boil. Reduce heat to low; cover and simmer 1½ hours, skimming fat as necessary.

Add remaining ingredients. Cover and cook 30 to 45 minutes more, or until meat is tender. Remove meat; cut into bite-size pieces. Add to soup. Makes 12 servings.

Per serving: 206 calories; 17 g. protein; 7 g. fat; 32% calories from fat; 50 mg. cholesterol; 19 g. carbohydrates; 354 mg. sodium; 3 g. fiber

Green Split Pea Soup

10   cups water
 1   package (16 ounces) green split peas, rinsed and
      drained
 1   ham hock
12   green onions, sliced with ½ tops also sliced
 1   cup diced carrots
 1   cup diced celery
 1   slice lemon
 1   bay leaf
 ½   teaspoon white or black pepper
     Salt to taste

In large saucepot or Dutch oven over high heat, combine all ingredients. Bring to boil. Reduce heat to low; simmer, uncovered, for 2 hours, or until peas are tender. Stir frequently. Add more water as needed.

Remove and discard lemon and bay leaf. Remove ham hock; chop edible ham coarsely. Return to soup. Makes 8 servings.

Per serving: 328 calories; 24 g. protein; 1 g. fat; 5% calories from fat; 7 mg. cholesterol; 55 g. carbohydrates; 223 mg. sodium; 13 g. fiber

Mushroom-Barley Soup

3   cups (about ½ pound) sliced mushrooms
½   cup chopped onions
½   cup chopped green peppers
⅓   cup butter or margarine
⅓   cup all-purpose flour
3   cups water
2   cups skim milk
½   cup quick-cooking barley
2   teaspoons Worcestershire sauce
1½ teaspoons salt
1   teaspoon dried parsley flakes
    Pepper to taste

Heat butter or margarine in large saucepot over medium heat. Sauté mushrooms, onions and green peppers. Blend in flour; cook, stirring, until flour is browned. Gradually stir in water and milk. Add remaining ingredients. Bring to boil. Reduce heat to low; cover and simmer 10 to 12 minutes, or until barley is tender. Makes 12 servings.

Note: Thin with additional milk or water if soup becomes too thick upon standing.

Per serving: 96 calories; 2 g. protein; 5 g. fat; 49% calories from fat; 14 mg. cholesterol; 10 g. carbohydrates; 334 mg. sodium; 1 g. fiber

Vegetarian Chowder

1   package (16 ounces) dried white beans (large or
      baby limas, navy beans or Great Northerns),
      rinsed and picked over
8   cups hot water
1½ teaspoons salt
1½ cups chopped celery
1   cup chopped onions
¼   cup butter or margarine
¼   cup all-purpose flour
⅛   teaspoon pepper
3   cups skim milk
1   can (16 ounces) tomatoes
1   can (12 ounces) vacuum-packed whole-kernel corn
1   cup (4 ounces) shredded Monterey Jack or sharp
      Cheddar cheese

In large saucepot or Dutch oven over high heat, place beans, water and salt. Bring to boil. Reduce heat to low; cover and cook until tender (about 1 hour for limas, about 2 to 2½ hours for navy and Great Northerns). Don't drain.

Heat butter or margarine in medium saucepan over medium heat. Sauté celery and onions. Stir in flour and pepper. Gradually stir in milk; bring to boil, stirring. Add to beans with remaining ingredients. Heat through. Makes 12 servings.

Note: For extra zip, add a few dashes of hot pepper sauce.

Per serving: 278 calories; 14 g. protein; 8 g. fat; 26% calories from fat; 21 mg. cholesterol; 39 g. carbohydrates; 286 mg. sodium; 12 g. fiber

Winter Spinach Soup

5   cups water
1   medium carrot, shredded
¼   cup medium barley
¼   cup dried lentils
¼   cup dried green split peas
¼   cup chopped onions
1   tablespoon dried parsley
2   teaspoons salt
    Pepper to taste
2   cups skim milk
1   package (10 ounces) frozen chopped spinach, thawed
2   tablespoons butter or margarine
¼   teaspoon ground nutmeg
1   hard cooked egg, chopped (optional)

In large saucepot or Dutch oven over high heat, place water, carrots, barley, lentils, peas, onions, parsley, salt and pepper. Bring to boil. Reduce heat to low; cover and simmer, stirring occasionally, 1 hour, or until beans are tender.

Add milk, spinach, butter or margarine and nutmeg. Heat through (do not boil). Top with chopped egg, if desired. Makes 8 servings.

Per serving: 110 calories; 6 g. protein; 3 g. fat; 25% calories from fat; 627 mg. cholesterol; 15 g. carbohydrates; 627 mg. sodium; 3 g. fiber

Lentil Soup

8 cups vegetable stock or water
1 package (16 ounces) lentils, rinsed
2 bay leaves
¼ cup canola, peanut, soybean or sunflower oil
1 medium onion, finely chopped
1 large rib celery with leaves, chopped
1 large carrot, coarsely shredded
1 small zucchini, coarsely shredded
2 cloves garlic, minced
2 tablespoons minced fresh parsley, or 2 teaspoons
    dried parsley
1 teaspoon dried thyme
1½ cups tomato juice
¼ cup red wine vinegar
1 teaspoon salt or to taste
    Shredded reduced-fat Cheddar cheese (optional)

In large saucepot or Dutch oven over high heat, place stock or water, lentils and bay leaves. Bring to boil. Reduce heat to low; cover and simmer for 1 to 1½ hours, or until lentils are almost tender.

Heat oil in small skillet over medium heat. Sauté onions until tender. Add celery, carrots, zucchini, garlic, parsley and thyme. Cook 5 minutes. Add to lentils with tomato juice, vinegar and salt. Cover and simmer 30 minutes. Top with cheese, if desired. Makes 6 servings.

Per serving: 332 calories; 19 g. protein; 9 g. fat; 26% calories from fat; 0 mg. cholesterol; 45 g. carbohydrates; 606 mg. sodium; 10 g. fiber

Chicken-Spinach Soup

1   broiler-fryer chicken (about 3 pounds), cut into
     quarters and skinned
6   quarts water
2   cups diced carrots
2   cups diced celery
1   cup diced onions
¼   cup chopped fresh parsley
3   packages (10 ounces each) frozen chopped spinach,
     thawed
1   package (10 ounces) frozen peas
4   eggs, lightly beaten
     Salt and pepper to taste
     Grated Parmesan cheese (optional)

In large saucepot or Dutch oven over high heat, place chicken and water. Bring to boil, skimming top as necessary. Reduce heat to low; cover and simmer 40 to 45 minutes, or until chicken is tender. Remove chicken from broth; cool slightly and remove from bones. Cut into bite-size pieces; set aside.

To broth, add carrots, celery, onions and parsley; cook 20 minutes. Add spinach and peas; cook 15 minutes. Add reserved chicken. Heat through. Remove from heat. Stirring constantly, gradually add eggs. Season with salt and pepper. Top with cheese, if desired. Makes 20 servings.

Per serving: 146 calories; 18 g. protein; 5 g. fat; 31% calories from fat; 100 mg. cholesterol; 6 g. carbohydrates; 124 mg. sodium; 2 g. fiber

Cauliflower Soup

2   cups chicken broth or stock
1   medium cauliflower (about 1¼ pounds), cut into
      small florets
2   cups skim milk
¼   cup butter or margarine, melted
2   tablespoons all-purpose flour
     Grated nutmeg to taste
     Salt to taste

In large saucepan over high heat, bring broth or stock to boil. Reduce heat to low; add cauliflower florets. Cook gently for 7 minutes. With slotted spoon, remove florets from liquid; set aside.

Add milk to liquid. Bring to boil. Reduce heat to low; whisk in butter or margarine and flour. Simmer 5 minutes. Season with nutmeg and salt. Add reserved florets. Makes 4 servings.

Per serving: 198 calories; 9 g. protein; 12 g. fat; 55% calories from fat; 33 mg. cholesterol; 13 g. carbohydrates; 568 mg. sodium; 3 g. fiber

SUPER SALADS

Florida Chicken Salad

¼   cup light mayonnaise
2   tablespoons lime juice
¼   teaspoon salt
⅛   teaspoon pepper
1   can (16 ounces) grapefruit sections, well drained
2   cups diced cooked chicken
1   cup diced celery
6   cups assorted salad greens
    Additional grapefruit sections for garnish (optional)

In large bowl, mix mayonnaise, lime juice, salt and pepper. Add grapefruit, chicken and celery. Toss gently to evenly coat. To serve, line bowl with greens and top with chicken salad and extra grapefruit sections, if desired. Makes 6 servings.

Per serving: 172 calories; 14 g. protein; 7 g. fat; 36% calories from fat; 45 mg. cholesterol; 12 g. carbohydrates; 229 mg. sodium; 2 g. fiber

Tuna-Rice Salad

1   cup uncooked rice
1   can (7 ounces) solid white tuna, drained
1½   cups finely chopped carrots
1   cup finely chopped celery
3   green onions, finely sliced
1   medium green pepper, finely chopped
1   pimiento, diced (optional)
¼   cup sweet pickle relish
¾   cup light mayonnaise
½   cup fresh parsley, chopped
¼   cup canola, corn, cottonseed, soybean or safflower oil
¼   cup cider vinegar
¼   teaspoon pepper
     Sliced tomatoes for garnish (optional)

Cook rice according to package directions; cool. In large bowl, place rice, tuna, carrots, celery, onions, green peppers, pimientos, if desired, and relish. Mix well. In small bowl, mix mayonnaise, ⅓ cup parsley, oil, vinegar and pepper. Pour over tuna mixture; toss gently to evenly coat.

Into 2-quart bowl, sprinkle remaining parsley. Spoon tuna-rice mixture into prepared bowl, pressing down. Chill thoroughly. To serve, run a knife around edge and turn out onto serving platter. Place sliced tomatoes around edge, if desired. Makes 8 servings.

Per serving: 289 calories; 8 g. protein; 16 g. fat; 51% calories from fat; 11 mg. cholesterol; 26 g. carbohydrates; 326 mg. sodium; 2 g. fiber

Oriental Salad

2   pounds skinless, boneless chicken breasts, cut into
       1-inch-wide strips
4   tablespoons soy sauce
⅔   cup canola, corn, cottonseed, soybean or safflower oil
1   clove garlic, scored
1   teaspoon shredded lemon peel
¼   cup lemon juice
1   bag (10 ounces) fresh spinach, washed and well
       drained
½   head iceberg lettuce, torn into bite-size pieces
3   cups fresh or canned bean sprouts, rinsed and well
       drained
¼   cup toasted sesame seeds
     Salt to taste

In small bowl or plastic bag, place chicken, 1 tablespoon soy sauce, 2 tablespoons oil, garlic and ½ teaspoon lemon peel; chill for several hours.

Divide chicken mixture into 3 batches. Heat 2 tablespoons oil in large skillet or wok over high heat. Place ⅓ chicken mixture in hot oil. Cook, stirring, 3 to 5 minutes until chicken is firm; remove to bowl. Repeat with next 2 batches of chicken. Discard garlic.

To chicken, add remaining soy sauce, oil, lemon peel and lemon juice. Toss gently until evenly coated. Chill. In large salad bowl, toss chicken mixture with spinach, lettuce, bean sprouts, sesame seeds and salt. Serve immediately. Makes 8 servings.

Per serving: 201 calories; 30 g. protein; 6 g. fat; 28% calories from fat; 71 mg. cholesterol; 6 g. carbohydrates; 613 mg. sodium; 3 g. fiber

Curried Chicken Salad

3	tablespoons instant minced onions
3	tablespoons water
2	tablespoons butter or margarine
1¼	teaspoons curry powder
¾	cup light mayonnaise
1	tablespoon lemon juice
½	teaspoon salt
	Dash cayenne pepper
3	cups diced cooked chicken
1	can (20 ounces) pineapple chunks, drained
1	red apple, cored and diced
2	tablespoons coarsely chopped nuts
⅓	cup golden raisins
4-6	lettuce leaves
2	tablespoons shredded or flaked coconut

In small bowl, mix onions and water; let stand 10 minutes. Melt butter or margarine in small skillet over medium heat. Add onions and curry powder; cook, stirring, 3 to 5 minutes. Set aside to cool.

In large bowl, stir curry mixture, mayonnaise, lemon juice, salt and pepper until well combined. Add chicken, pineapple, apples, nuts and raisins; toss gently to evenly coat. To serve, line salad bowl with lettuce; fill with chicken salad. Sprinkle with coconut. Makes 6 servings.

Note: Cooked turkey may be substituted for chicken.

Per serving: 368 calories; 21 g. protein; 21 g. fat; 52% calories from fat; 82 mg. cholesterol; 23 g. carbohydrates; 507 mg. sodium; 2 g. fiber

Potato-Brussels Salad

1   cup Brussels sprouts
1   tablespoon nonfat plain yogurt
1   tablespoon light mayonnaise
1   tablespoon orange juice
¼   cup chopped fresh parsley
    Salt and pepper to taste
1   large orange, peeled and sectioned
1   pound potatoes, peeled, cooked and diced

In small saucepan over medium heat, cook Brussels sprouts in salted water 5 minutes, or until tender. Drain. Cool and slice.

In large bowl, stir yogurt, mayonnaise, orange juice, parsley, salt and pepper until well blended. Reserve a few orange sections for garnish. Add remaining orange sections, Brussels sprouts and potatoes; toss gently to evenly coat. Cover and chill several hours. To serve, top with reserved orange sections. Makes 6 servings.

Per serving: 91 calories; 2 g. protein; 1 g. fat; 10% calories from fat; 0 mg. cholesterol; 19 g. carbohydrates; 27 mg. sodium; 3 g. fiber

Wintery Turkey Salad

2 cups coarsely chopped cooked turkey
½ cup light mayonnaise
¼ cup thinly sliced celery
2 tablespoons finely chopped pimientos
2 tablespoons drained capers
1 tablespoon finely chopped green onions
1 tablespoon finely chopped parsley
1 tablespoon lemon juice or to taste
1 teaspoon Dijon mustard
  Salt to taste
  Few drops hot-pepper sauce
  Bibb lettuce for garnish (optional)

In large bowl, place all ingredients except lettuce; toss gently to evenly coat. Serve on bed of lettuce, if desired. Makes 4 servings.

Per serving: 223 calories; 20 g. protein; 13 g. fat; 56% calories from fat; 63 mg. cholesterol; 3 g. carbohydrates; 835 mg. sodium; 0 g. fiber

Molded Vegetable Salad

1   package (4-serving size) lemon, lime or orange gelatin
¾   teaspoon salt
1   cup boiling water
¾   cup cold water
¼   cup finely chopped green peppers
2   tablespoons cider vinegar
2   teaspoons grated onions
    Ground pepper to taste
¾   cup finely chopped cabbage
¾   cup finely chopped celery
2   tablespoons diced pimientos

In medium bowl, place gelatin and salt. Pour in boiling water; stir until dissolved. Stir in cold water, green peppers, vinegar, onions and pepper. Chill until slightly thickened, about 1½ hours. Fold in cabbage, celery and pimiento; pour into 1-quart mold. Chill until firm, about 4 hours. Makes 6 servings.

Note: Equal quantities of diced tomatoes, cucumbers, shredded carrots, stuffed olives and/or thin onion rings may be substituted for the vegetables.

Per serving: 60 calories; 1 g. protein; 0 g. fat; 1% calories from fat; 0 mg. cholesterol; 14 g. carbohydrates; 317 mg. sodium; 0 g. fiber

Health Salad

1 head Boston lettuce, rinsed
1 small cucumber, thinly sliced
2 small tomatoes, peeled and sliced
1 medium green pepper, sliced
½ large avocado, peeled and sliced
5 radishes, sliced
1 medium peach, peeled and cubed
6 thin slices pineapple
½ can (11 ounces) mandarin orange segments
1 pint strawberries, hulled
  Fat-free dressing (optional)

On large serving platter or in salad bowl, tear lettuce into bite-size pieces. Top with arrangement of remaining ingredients. Serve with dressing, if desired. Makes 6 servings.

Per serving: 73 calories; 2 g. protein; 3 g. fat; 33% calories from fat; 0 mg. cholesterol; 12 g. carbohydrates; 9 mg. sodium; 5 g. fiber

Spinach Salad Veronique

4 cups torn fresh spinach leaves
½ small red onion, thinly sliced
½ cup thinly sliced seedless green grapes
4 tablespoons fat-free Italian dressing
1 tablespoon chopped fresh mint leaves for garnish
(optional)

In each of 2 salad bowls, place 2 cups spinach; top with onions and grapes. Top each with 2 tablespoons dressing. Garnish with mint, if desired. Makes 2 servings.

Per serving: 71 calories; 4 g. protein; 0 g. fat; 8% calories from fat; 0 mg. cholesterol; 15 g. carbohydrates; 235 mg. sodium; 5 g. fiber

Red Cabbage and Apple Salad

½ small red cabbage, finely shredded
3 Delicious or Golden Delicious apples, cored and
coarsely shredded
¼-⅓ cup fat-free French dressing

In large bowl, place cabbage and apples. Add dressing; toss to evenly coat. Makes 4 servings.

Per serving: 118 calories; 1 g. protein; 0 g. fat; 5% calories from fat; 0 mg. cholesterol; 29 g. carbohydrates; 154 mg. sodium; 5 g. fiber

Fruit Slaw

¼ cup light mayonnaise
1 tablespoon pineapple juice
¼ teaspoon salt
4 cups shredded cabbage
3 medium oranges, peeled and cut into sections
⅓ cup drained crushed pineapple
½ cup chopped green peppers

In large bowl, mix mayonnaise, pineapple juice and salt until well blended. Add cabbage, orange sections, pineapple and green peppers; toss gently until evenly coated. Makes 6 servings.

Per serving: 80 calories; 1 g. protein; 3 g. fat; 37% calories from fat; 3 mg. cholesterol; 12 g. carbohydrates; 174 mg. sodium; 3 g. fiber

Zucchini Salad

6 medium zucchini, thinly sliced
1 large onion, sliced
1 clove garlic, sliced
   Fat-free French dressing
3 large tomatoes, thinly sliced
   Lettuce leaves
   Parmesan cheese for garnish (optional)

In large saucepan over medium heat, cook zucchini in salted water 2 to 3 minutes; drain well. In large bowl, place zucchini, onions and garlic; cover with French dressing. Cover and chill overnight.

To serve, drain zucchini; discard onions and garlic. On large platter, arrange tomato slices over bed of lettuce; top with zucchini. Garnish with cheese, if desired. Makes 6 servings.

Per serving: 48 calories; 2 g. protein; 0 g. fat; 7% calories from fat; 0 mg. cholesterol; 10 g. carbohydrates; 154 mg. sodium; 3 g. fiber

Lima Bean Salad

2   cans (17 ounces each) lima beans
¾   cup wine vinegar
1   clove garlic, minced
¼   cup finely minced onions
¼   cup chopped fresh parsley
2   tablespoons sugar
½   teaspoon salt
¼   teaspoon pepper

Drain lima beans, reserving ⅔ cup bean liquid. In large bowl, mix reserved bean liquid, vinegar, garlic, onions, parsley, sugar, salt and pepper until well blended. Add lima beans; toss gently to evenly coat. Cover and chill several hours. Makes 4 servings.

Per serving: 214 calories; 11 g. protein; 0 g. fat; 2% calories from fat; 0 mg. cholesterol; 43 g. carbohydrates; 1030 mg. sodium; 16 g. fiber

Layered Vegetable Salad

1 package (10 ounces) frozen baby lima beans
2 cups fresh cauliflower florets, cut into bite-size pieces
1 small red onion, thinly sliced
1 cup alfalfa sprouts
1 cup fresh broccoli or broccoflower florets, cut into
   bite-size pieces
1 cup (4 ounces) shredded reduced-fat Cheddar cheese
2 tablespoons chopped walnuts
   Fat-free Italian dressing (optional)

In small saucepan over medium heat, cook lima beans in salted water 5 minutes; drain. In medium glass salad bowl, place ½ each lima beans and cauliflower, onions, sprouts, and broccoli or broccoflower. Repeat layers using remaining vegetables. Top with cheese and walnuts. To serve, toss gently and, if desired, top with dressing. Makes 6 servings.

Per serving: 130 calories; 10 g. protein; 4 g. fat; 31% calories from fat; 6 mg. cholesterol; 14 g. carbohydrates; 156 mg. sodium; 6 g. fiber

Dilled Cucumber and Yogurt Salad

1   cup water
¼   cup cider or white vinegar
1   slice onion
1   teaspoon dried dill
2   cucumbers, thinly sliced
1   cup nonfat plain yogurt
½   teaspoon salt
⅛   teaspoon turmeric
     Dash pepper
¼   cup diced cooked potatoes
4   cups torn leafy lettuce or mixed greens

In large bowl, place water, vinegar, onion and dill. Add cucumber slices; let stand at least 30 minutes. Discard onion and drain well.

In serving bowl, mix yogurt, salt, turmeric and pepper. Add cucumbers and potatoes; toss gently to evenly coat. On serving platter, arrange lettuce or greens; top with cucumber mixture. Makes 4 servings.

Per serving: 60 calories; 5 g. protein; 0 g. fat; 6% calories from fat; 1 mg. cholesterol; 10 g. carbohydrates; 316 mg. sodium; 2 g. fiber

Carrot Salad

2 cans (16 ounces each) sliced carrots, drained
1 small onion, finely chopped
1 medium pepper, finely chopped
3 ribs celery, finely chopped
1 cup undiluted condensed tomato soup
1 cup sugar
¾ cup cider vinegar
¼ cup canola, corn, cottonseed, safflower or soybean oil
1 tablespoon dry mustard
1 tablespoon Worcestershire sauce
   Lettuce leaves for garnish (optional)

In large bowl, place carrots, onions, peppers and celery; set aside. In small saucepan over high heat, mix tomato soup, sugar, vinegar, oil, mustard and Worcestershire sauce. Bring to boil, stirring until smooth. Pour over carrot mixture. Cool slightly. Cover and chill overnight. Serve over lettuce, if desired. Makes 10 servings.

Per serving: 179 calories; 1 g. protein; 6 g. fat; 30% calories from fat; 0 mg. cholesterol; 31 g. carbohydrates; 482 mg. sodium; 1 g. fiber

Spicy Lentil Salad

2   cups dry lentils, rinsed and picked over
3   cloves garlic, peeled
2   hot red or green chili peppers, seeded and chopped
4   tablespoons olive oil
1   teaspoon salt
3-6   tablespoons cider vinegar
½   cup finely chopped onions
    Pepper to taste

In large saucepot over high heat, place lentils and enough water to cover. Bring to boil. Reduce heat to low; add garlic and chili peppers. Cover and simmer 20 to 30 minutes, or until lentils are tender. Discard garlic; drain well.

In large bowl, mix cooked lentils, oil and salt; cover and chill 2 hours. Just before serving, stir in vinegar, onions and peppers until well blended. Makes 6 servings.

Per serving: 306 calories; 18 g. protein; 9 g. fat; 27% calories from fat; 0 mg. cholesterol; 39 g. carbohydrates; 363 mg. sodium; 8 g. fiber

Garbanzo Bean Salad

1   can (15 to 19 ounces) garbanzo beans (chickpeas),
    drained
3   green onions, chopped
¾   cup chopped celery
½   cup sliced pitted green olives
¼   cup chopped pimientos
2   tablespoons olive oil
2   tablespoons tarragon vinegar
½   teaspoon salt
¼   teaspoon garlic powder
    Dash of pepper
    Lettuce for garnish (optional)

In medium bowl, place all ingredients except lettuce; toss gently to evenly coat. Cover and chill 24 hours. Serve in lettuce cups, if desired. Makes 4 servings.

Per serving: 225 calories; 8 g. protein; 11 g. fat; 44% calories from fat; 0 mg. cholesterol; 25 g. carbohydrates; 675 mg. sodium; 7 g. fiber

Garden Pea Salad

1	package (10 ounces) frozen peas
¼	cup canola, corn, cottonseed, safflower or soybean oil
2½	tablespoons cider vinegar
¾	teaspoon salt
¼	teaspoon dried thyme
⅛	teaspoon pepper
1	cup alfalfa sprouts
½	cup (2 ounces) cubed reduced-fat Cheddar cheese
¼	cup chopped celery
¼	cup coarsely chopped unsalted cashews
2	tablespoons nonfat plain yogurt
1	tablespoon light mayonnaise

In small saucepan over medium heat, place ½ cup water and peas. Bring to boil. Remove from heat; let stand 1 or 2 minutes, or just until peas are heated through. Drain; place in medium bowl.

In small bowl, mix oil, vinegar, salt, thyme and pepper; pour over peas. Cover and chill several hours. Just before serving, drain off marinade; add remaining ingredients. Toss gently to evenly coat. Makes 6 servings.

Per serving: 128 calories; 6 g. protein; 7 g. fat; 52% calories from fat; 4 mg. cholesterol; 9 g. carbohydrates; 179 mg. sodium; 3 g. fiber

Confetti Salad

2   cups cooked mixed vegetables
½   cup shredded carrots
½   cup chopped celery
¼   cup chopped green peppers
1   tablespoon minced onions
¼   cup fat-free French dressing
¼   cup crumbled Roquefort or blue cheese
    Lettuce for garnish (optional)

In medium bowl, place mixed vegetables, carrots, celery, peppers and onions. Add dressing; stir until well mixed. Add cheese; toss gently to evenly coat. Cover and chill several hours. To serve, toss again and place in lettuce cups, if desired. Makes 4 servings.

Per serving: 93 calories; 4 g. protein; 2 g. fat; 20% calories from fat; 5 mg. cholesterol; 15 g. carbohydrates; 294 mg. sodium; 4 g. fiber

Grapefruit Salad

2   large firm grapefruits
2   tablespoons light mayonnaise
1   tablespoon nonfat sour cream
2   teaspoons lemon juice
1   teaspoon thawed frozen orange juice concentrate
⅛   teaspoon paprika
1   cup diced cooked potatoes
½   cup diced unpeeled cucumbers
     Parsley for garnish (optional)

With sharp knife, slice top off grapefruit. Remove grapefruit sections, keeping them intact; drain sections and set aside. Cut design in edge of grapefruit shell with kitchen shears as desired. If necessary, slice small amount off bottom of grapefruit to keep in upright position.

In medium bowl, stir mayonnaise, sour cream, lemon juice, orange juice concentrate and paprika. Add reserved grapefruit sections, potatoes and cucumbers. Toss gently to evenly coat. Cover and chill several hours. To serve, spoon into grapefruit shells. Top with parsley, if desired. Makes 2 servings.

Per serving: 260 calories; 4 g. protein; 5 g. fat; 18% calories from fat; 6 mg. cholesterol; 50 g. carbohydrates; 132 mg. sodium; 5 g. fiber

Tabbouleh Salad

1   cup bulgur (cracked wheat)
1½ cups boiling water
1   bunch parsley, finely chopped
2   medium tomatoes, peeled and finely chopped
1   large cucumber, finely chopped
¼   cup lemon juice
¼   cup olive oil
12 chopped fresh mint leaves, or 2 tablespoons dried
      mint leaves
½   teaspoon garlic salt
      Salt and pepper to taste

In large bowl, place bulgur and boiling water; let stand 2 hours. Drain well.

In large bowl, place soaked bulgur and remaining ingredients. Toss until well blended. Cover and chill several hours. Makes 8 servings.

Note: May be made a day ahead.

Per serving: 149 calories; 3 g. protein; 7 g. fat; 42% calories from fat; 0 mg. cholesterol; 19 g. carbohydrates; 37 mg. sodium; 5 g. fiber

BOUNTIFUL BREADS

Basic Muffins

2   cups all-purpose flour
⅓   cup sugar
1   tablespoon baking powder
1   teaspoon salt
1   egg
1   cup skim milk
⅓   cup canola, corn, safflower or soybean oil

Preheat oven to 400°F. Grease 12 (2½-inch) muffin cups well or line with paper baking cups. In large bowl, mix flour, sugar, baking powder and salt. In separate bowl, blend egg, milk and oil. Add to flour mixture all at once, stirring just until dry ingredients are moistened. Spoon into prepared muffin cups, filling each about halfway. Bake 20 to 25 minutes, or until muffins are lightly browned. Makes 12 muffins.

Per muffin: 158 calories; 3 g. protein; 6 g. fat; 35% calories from fat; 23 mg. cholesterol; 22 g. carbohydrates; 277 mg. sodium; trace g. fiber

VARIATIONS

Blueberry Muffins: Increase sugar to ½ cup. Lightly blend in ¾ cup fresh or drained canned blueberries when combining liquid and dry ingredients. Do not crush berries.

Per muffin: 176 calories; 3 g. protein; 6 g. fat; 32% calories from fat; 23 mg. cholesterol; 26 g. carbohydrates; 277 mg. sodium; 1 g. fiber

Oatmeal-Raisin Muffins: Reduce flour to 1¼ cups. Mix 1 cup quick-cooking rolled oats and 1½ cup raisins with dry ingredients before adding liquid.

Per muffin: 217 calories; 4 g. protein; 6 g. fat; 26% calories from fat; 23 mg. cholesterol; 37 g. carbohydrates; 279 mg. sodium; 2 g. fiber

Honey Corn Muffins

¾   cup sifted all-purpose flour
⅓   cup cornmeal
1¼   teaspoon baking powder
½   teaspoon salt
1   egg, well beaten
⅓   cup skim milk
¼   cup honey
3   tablespoons canola, corn, safflower or soybean oil
¼   cup peeled diced apple

Preheat oven to 400°F. Grease 8 (2-inch) muffin cups well or line with paper baking cups. In large bowl, mix flour, cornmeal, baking powder and salt. In separate bowl, blend egg, milk, honey and oil. Add to flour mixture all at once, stirring just until dry ingredients are moistened. Gently stir in apple. Spoon into prepared muffin cups. Bake 15 to 20 minutes, or until muffins are well browned. Makes 8 muffins.

Per muffin: 148 calories; 2 g. protein; 5 g. fat; 34% calories from fat; 34 mg. cholesterol; 22 g. carbohydrates; 220 mg. sodium; trace g. fiber

Nutty Carrot Muffins

1 cup whole-wheat pastry flour
¾ cup all-purpose flour
¼ cup firmly packed brown sugar
¼ cup nonfat dry milk powder
2½ teaspoons baking powder
1 teaspoon salt
⅔ cup water
⅓ cup canola, corn, safflower or soybean oil
1 egg
1 large carrot, cut into ½-inch slices
½ cup unsalted peanuts

Preheat oven to 400°F. Grease 12 (2½-inch) muffin cups well or line with paper baking cups. In large bowl, mix flours, sugar, dry milk, baking powder and salt. In blender, place remaining ingredients; blend until smooth. Add carrot-peanut mixture to flour mixture all at once, stirring just until dry ingredients are moistened. Spoon into prepared muffin cups. Bake 20 to 25 minutes, or until muffins are firm to touch. Serve warm. Makes 12 muffins.

Per muffin: 177 calories; 4 g. protein; 9 g. fat; 45% calories from fat; 23 mg. cholesterol; 20 g. carbohydrates; 265 mg. sodium; 2 g. fiber

Oatmeal Muffins

1   cup whole-wheat flour
¾   cup rolled oats
½   cup raisins or chopped prunes, figs, apricots or dates
¼   cup firmly packed light brown sugar
1   tablespoon baking powder
¾   teaspoon salt
½   teaspoon baking soda
¼   teaspoon nutmeg
1   egg, lightly beaten
1   cup skim milk
¼   cup canola, corn, safflower or soybean oil

Preheat oven to 400°F. Grease 12 (2½-inch) muffin cups well or line with paper baking cups. In large bowl, mix flour, oats, raisins or prunes, figs, apricots or dates, sugar, baking powder, salt, baking soda, and nutmeg. In separate bowl, blend egg, milk and oil. Add to flour mixture all at once, stirring just until dry ingredients are moistened. Spoon into prepared muffin cups, filling each about halfway. Bake 20 to 25 minutes, or until muffins are well browned. Makes 12 muffins.

Per muffin: 146 calories; 3 g. protein; 5 g. fat; 33% calories from fat; 23 mg. cholesterol; 21 g. carbohydrates; 136 mg. sodium; 2 g. fiber

Prune-Nugget Muffins

½ cup all-purpose flour
½ cup whole-wheat pastry flour
¼ cup wheat germ
2 teaspoons baking powder
1 teaspoon grated lemon peel
½ teaspoon salt
1 egg, lightly beaten
⅔ cup skim milk
¼ cup honey
¼ cup canola, corn, safflower or soybean oil
1 cup coarsely chopped prunes
⅓ cup chopped walnuts or pecans

Preheat oven to 400°F. Grease 12 (2½-inch) muffin cups well or line with paper baking cups. In large bowl, mix flours, wheat germ, baking powder, lemon peel and salt. In separate bowl, blend egg, milk, honey and oil. Add to flour mixture all at once, stirring just until dry ingredients are moistened. Gently stir in prunes and nuts. Spoon into prepared muffin cups. Bake 18 to 20 minutes, or until muffins are lightly browned. Makes 12 muffins.

Per muffin: 185 calories; 3 g. protein; 7 g. fat; 34% calories from fat; 23 mg. cholesterol; 28 g. carbohydrates; 158 mg. sodium; 3 g. fiber

Ginger Muffins

2 cups sifted all-purpose flour
⅔ cup sugar
1½ teaspoons baking soda
1½ teaspoons ground ginger
1½ teaspoons ground cinnamon
¼ teaspoon ground nutmeg
⅔ cup dark molasses
⅔ cup buttermilk
⅓ cup canola, corn, safflower or soybean oil
1 egg, slightly beaten

Preheat oven to 425°F. Grease 12 (2½-inch) muffin cups well or line with paper baking cups. In large bowl, mix flour, sugar, baking soda, ginger, cinnamon and nutmeg. In separate bowl, blend molasses, buttermilk, oil and egg. Add to flour mixture all at once, stirring just until dry ingredients are moistened. Spoon into prepared muffin cups. Bake 15 to 20 minutes, or until muffins are done. Makes 12 muffins.

Per muffin: 213 calories; 3 g. protein; 5 g. fat; 25% calories from fat; 23 mg. cholesterol; 37 g. carbohydrates; 140 mg. sodium; trace g. fiber

Applesauce-Banana Muffins

1 cup whole-wheat flour
⅔ cup all-purpose flour
2½ teaspoons baking powder
½ teaspoon salt
¾ cup unsweetened applesauce
1 very ripe small banana, mashed
1 egg
¼ cup canola, corn, safflower or soybean oil
½ cup raisins (optional)

Preheat oven to 375°F. Grease 12 (2½-inch) muffin cups well or line with paper baking cups. In large bowl, mix flours, baking powder and salt. In separate bowl, blend applesauce, banana, egg and oil. Add to flour mixture all at once, with raisins, if desired, stirring just until dry ingredients are moistened. Spoon into prepared muffin cups. Bake 20 to 25 minutes, or until muffins are golden brown. Serve warm. Makes 12 muffins.

Per muffin: 122 calories; 2 g. protein; 5 g. fat; 38% calories from fat; 22 mg. cholesterol; 16 g. carbohydrates; 164 mg. sodium; 2 g. fiber

Honey Rye Bread

2   envelopes dry active yeast
½   cup lukewarm (105-111°F) water
1½   cups lukewarm (105-111°F) milk
¼   cup honey
2   tablespoons butter, softened
3   teaspoons salt
3¼   cups medium rye flour
2½   cups all-purpose flour

Grease two 9 x 5-inch loaf pans; set aside. In large bowl, dissolve yeast in water. With wooden spoon, stir in milk, honey, butter, salt and 1¼ cups rye flour. Beat in more rye flour, 1 cup at a time, until mixture is smooth. Work in any remaining rye flour and all-purpose flour until dough leaves sides of bowl. Turn out on well-floured surface; knead 10 minutes until elastic. Place in greased bowl; turn dough to grease top. Cover; let rise in warm, draft-free place until doubled in bulk, 1 to 1½ hours. Punch down; turn out on well-floured surface.

Divide into two equal portions. Shape each portion into loaf, and place each into prepared loaf pans. Cover; let rise 1 to 1¼ hours until doubled. Bake in preheated 375°F oven 30 to 35 minutes. Turn out on wire racks to cool. Makes 2 loaves (15 slices each).

Per slice: 101 calories; 3 g. protein; 1 g. fat; 10% calories from fat; 2 mg. cholesterol; 20 g. carbohydrates; 227 mg. sodium; 2 g. fiber

Whole-Wheat Date Biscuits

2 cups whole-wheat flour
2 teaspoons baking powder
½ teaspoon salt
½ teaspoon ground cloves
4 tablespoons shortening or margarine
¾ cup finely chopped dates
½ cup finely chopped nuts (optional)
¾ cup skim milk

Preheat oven to 450°F. Grease large baking sheet; set aside. In large bowl, mix flour, baking powder, salt and cloves. With pastry blender or 2 knives used scissor fashion, cut in shortening or margarine until mixture resembles coarse cornmeal. Add dates; stir in nuts, if desired. Add milk, stirring just until ingredients are moistened. Turn out on lightly floured surface and knead briefly. Roll ¾ inch thick; with small biscuit cutter or glass, cut into rounds. Place on prepared baking sheet. Bake 15 minutes until golden brown. Makes 22 biscuits.

Per biscuit: 95 calories; 2 g. protein; 4 g. fat; 39% calories from fat; 0 mg. cholesterol; 13 g. carbohydrates; 83 mg. sodium; 2 g. fiber

Orange-Nut Bread

2 cups sifted all-purpose flour
¾ cup sifted whole-wheat flour
⅓ cup wheat germ
½ cup sugar
1 tablespoon baking powder
½ teaspoon baking soda
1 cup orange juice
⅓ cup canola, corn, safflower or soybean oil
1 egg, lightly beaten
⅓ cup walnuts, chopped
2 tablespoons shredded orange peel

Preheat oven to 350°F. Grease 9 x 5-inch loaf pan. In large bowl, mix flours, wheat germ, sugar, baking powder and baking soda. In separate bowl, blend orange juice, oil and egg. Add to flour mixture all at once with nuts and orange peel until well blended. Spoon into prepared pan. Bake 55 to 60 minutes, or until pick inserted into center comes out clean. Remove from pan to wire rack; cool completely. Makes 1 loaf (16 slices).

Per slice: 167 calories; 3 g. protein; 6 g. fat; 33% calories from fat; 17 mg. cholesterol; 24 g. carbohydrates; 92 mg. sodium; 1 g. fiber

Spoonbread

2 cups boiling water
1 cup yellow cornmeal
3 tablespoons butter
1 teaspoon salt
    Cholesterol-free, fat-free egg substitute, equivalent to
        3 eggs
1 cup skim milk

Preheat oven to 375°F. Grease 2-quart ovenproof casserole; set aside. In large bowl, place boiling water; slowly add cornmeal, stirring constantly until thick and smooth. Add butter and salt; cool to lukewarm. Add egg substitute and milk. Beat for 2 minutes; pour into prepared casserole. Bake 35 minutes, or until golden brown. Spoon out while piping hot. Serves 8.

Per serving: 123 calories; 4 g. protein; 4 g. fat; 34% calories from fat; 12 mg. cholesterol; 15 g. carbohydrates; 356 mg. sodium; 1 g. fiber

Steamed Brown Bread

1   cup medium rye flour
1   cup whole-wheat flour
1   cup cornmeal
2   teaspoons baking soda
1   teaspoon salt
2   cups buttermilk or sour 1% low-fat milk
¾   cup molasses
1   cup raisins

Grease two 1-pound coffee cans; set aside. In large bowl, mix flours, cornmeal, baking soda and salt. In separate bowl, blend milk and molasses. Add to flour mixture, stirring until well blended. Stir in raisins. Spoon evenly into prepared cans. Tightly cover cans with waxed paper.

In large saucepot, place wire rack and enough water to just cover rack. Place cans on rack; cover saucepot tightly. Steam over low heat 3 hours. Makes 2 loaves (12 slices each).

Per slice: 104 calories; 2 g. protein; 0 g. fat; 4% calories from fat; 0 mg. cholesterol; 23 g. carbohydrates; 189 mg. sodium; 2 g. fiber

Molasses Brown Bread

2   tablespoons lemon juice
2   cups skim milk
1   cup all-purpose flour
1   cup whole-wheat flour
1   cup cornmeal
2   teaspoons baking soda
1   teaspoon salt
¾   cup unsulfured molasses
¾   cup diced candied fruit, raisins or nuts (optional)

Preheat oven to 350°F. Grease four 16-ounce cans or three 20-ounce cans; set aside. Add lemon juice to milk; set aside at least 5 minutes.

In large bowl, mix flours, cornmeal, baking soda and salt. In another bowl, blend milk mixture and molasses. Add to flour mixture, stirring just until dry ingredients are moistened. Stir in candied fruit, raisins or nuts, if desired. Spoon mixture evenly into prepared cans. Bake 45 to 50 minutes, or until pick inserted near center comes out clean. Cool in cans 10 minutes; turn out onto wire rack. Serve warm, if desired. Makes 3 or 4 loaves (24 servings).

Per serving: 108 calories; 2 g. protein; 0 g. fat; 2% calories from fat; 0 mg. cholesterol; 24 g. carbohydrates; 190 mg. sodium; 1 g. fiber

Corn Bread

1 cup cornmeal
1 cup all-purpose flour
4 teaspoons baking powder
1 tablespoon sugar
½ teaspoon salt
1½ cups skim milk
1 egg
¼ cup canola, corn, safflower or soybean oil

Preheat oven to 450°F. Grease 8 x 8-inch baking pan. In large bowl, mix cornmeal, flour, baking powder, sugar and salt. In separate bowl, blend milk, egg and oil. Add to flour mixture all at once, stirring until well blended. Spoon into prepared baking pan. Bake 25 to 30 minutes, or until golden brown. Makes 12 servings.

Per serving: 139 calories; 3 g. protein; 5 g. fat; 35% calories from fat; 23 mg. cholesterol; 18 g. carbohydrates; 220 mg. sodium; 1 g. fiber

Zucchini Bread

2 cups whole-wheat flour
¼ cup wheat germ
¼ cup unprocessed bran
3½ teaspoons ground cinnamon
1 teaspoon baking soda
¼ teaspoon baking powder
  Cholesterol-free, fat-free egg substitute, equivalent to
    3 eggs
1 cup honey
1 cup canola, corn, safflower or soybean oil
2 teaspoons vanilla extract
2 cups shredded, unpeeled zucchini
¾ cup chopped walnuts or pecans
½ cup raisins (optional)

Preheat oven to 325°F. Grease two 8½ x 4½-inch loaf pans. In large bowl, mix flour, wheat germ, bran, cinnamon, baking soda and baking powder. In separate bowl, blend egg substitute, honey, oil and vanilla. Add with zucchini and nuts to flour mixture all at once, stirring until blended. Stir in raisins, if desired. Spoon into prepared loaf pans. Bake 60 to 70 minutes, or until pick inserted into center comes out clean. Makes 2 loaves (12 slices each).

Per slice: 201 calories; 3 g. protein; 11 g. fat; 50% calories from fat; 0 mg. cholesterol; 23 g. carbohydrates; 52 mg. sodium; 2 g. fiber

Nutty Brown Bread

1   cup all-purpose flour
1   cup whole-wheat flour
½   cup firmly packed light brown sugar
½   cup walnuts, finely grated (makes about ¾ cup)
2   teaspoons baking powder
¾   teaspoon salt
¼   teaspoon baking soda
1   egg
1¼ cups skim milk

Preheat oven to 350°F. Grease 8½ x 4½-inch loaf pan. In large bowl, mix flours, sugar, walnuts, baking powder, salt and baking soda. In separate bowl, blend egg and milk. Add to flour mixture all at once, stirring just until dry ingredients are moistened. Spoon into prepared loaf pan. Bake 50 minutes, or until pick inserted into center comes out clean. (Top will have crack.) Turn out on wire rack; cool completely right side up. Makes 1 loaf (12 slices).

Note: Inexpensive rotary-type, hand-operated grater works well for grating nuts.

Per slice: 154 calories; 4 g. protein; 4 g. fat; 22% calories from fat; 23 mg. cholesterol; 26 g. carbohydrates; 229 mg. sodium; 2 g. fiber

Easy Whole-Wheat Bread

1   envelope dry active yeast
1   teaspoon salt
1   teaspoon honey
3   cups fairly hot (120-130°F) water
4   cups whole-wheat flour
½-1 cup wheat flakes, rye flakes, rolled oats or wheat germ

Preheat oven to 400°F. Grease 9 x 5-inch loaf pan; set aside. In large bowl, place yeast, salt and honey. Pour in water; let stand until surface is bubbly. Stir in flour and enough flakes, oats or wheat germ to make thick yet softer, more liquid bread dough. Place dough in loaf pan; let stand in warm, draft-free place 10 minutes. Bake 45 minutes, or until loaf sounds hollow when lightly tapped. Makes 1 loaf (12 slices).

Per slice: 164 calories; 6 g. protein; 1 g. fat; 9% calories from fat; 0 mg. cholesterol; 33 g. carbohydrates; 190 mg. sodium; 5 g. fiber

Whole-Wheat Irish Soda Bread

4   cups whole-wheat flour
1   tablespoon baking powder
2   teaspoons salt
½   teaspoon baking soda
2   cups buttermilk

Preheat oven to 350°F. Grease large baking sheet; set side. In large bowl, mix flour, baking powder, salt and baking soda. Add buttermilk, stirring to form soft dough. Turn out on floured surface; knead lightly for 1 minute. Shape into two flat, round patties, about 8 inches in diameter. Slash large cross in each top. Place on prepared baking sheet. Bake 40 minutes, or until bread sounds hollow when lightly tapped. Cool 5 minutes on wire rack before cutting. Makes 2 loaves (12 slices each).

Per slice: 75 calories; 3 g. protein; 0 g. fat; 7% calories from fat; 0 mg. cholesterol; 15 g. carbohydrates; 258 mg. sodium; 2 g. fiber

Banana Bread

¾ cup sugar
½ cup shortening
Cholesterol-free, fat-free egg substitute, equivalent to
   2 eggs
1 cup mashed banana
1¾ cups all-purpose flour
2 teaspoons baking powder
½ teaspoon baking soda
½ teaspoon salt

Preheat oven to 350°F. Grease 9 x 5-inch loaf pan; set aside. In large bowl with mixer, beat sugar, shortening and egg substitute until light and well combined. Stir in banana. Stir in flour, baking powder, baking soda and salt just until smooth. Spoon into prepared pan. Bake 50 to 60 minutes, or until firm when lightly touched on top. Cool in pan on wire rack 10 minutes. Remove and cool completely. Makes 1 loaf (16 slices).

Per slice: 160 calories; 2 g. protein; 6 g. fat; 37% calories from fat; 0 mg. cholesterol; 23 g. carbohydrates; 147 mg. sodium; trace g. fiber

VARIATION

Orange-Banana Bread: Add 1 tablespoon grated orange peel to sugar-egg mixture.

Per slice: 160 calories; 2 g. protein; 6 g. fat; 37% calories from fat; 0 mg. cholesterol; 23 g. carbohydrates; 147 mg. sodium; trace g. fiber

Apricot Bran Loaf

1   cup dried apricots, cut into small pieces
½   cup plus 2 tablespoons sugar
1½ cups sifted all-purpose flour
4   teaspoons baking powder
½   teaspoon salt
1½ cups whole-bran cereal
1   cup skim milk
    Cholesterol-free, fat-free egg substitute equivalent to
       2 eggs
⅓   cup canola, corn, safflower or soybean oil

Preheat oven to 350°F. Grease 9 x 5-inch loaf pan; set aside. In medium bowl, place apricots in enough boiling water to cover; let stand 10 minutes. Drain; stir in 2 tablespoons sugar and set aside.

In large bowl, mix remaining ½ cup sugar, flour, baking powder and salt. In separate bowl, blend cereal, milk, egg substitute and oil. Add to flour mixture all at once, stirring just until dry ingredients are moistened. Stir in apricot mixture. Spoon into prepared loaf pan. Bake 60 minutes, or until pick inserted into center comes out clean. Remove from pan; cool completely on wire rack. Makes 1 loaf (16 slices).

Note: Dried pears, prunes or apples may be substituted for apricots.

Per slice: 156 calories; 4 g. protein; 5 g. fat; 28% calories from fat; 34 mg. cholesterol; 26 g. carbohydrates; 257 mg. sodium; 3 g. fiber

EXCITING ENTRÉES

Vegetable-Stuffed Green Peppers

4   medium green peppers
1   cup drained canned corn or thawed frozen whole-
    kernel corn
¾   cup diced tomatoes
½   cup soft bread crumbs
¼   cup finely chopped celery
    Cholesterol-free, fat-free egg substitute, equivalent to
        2 eggs
2   tablespoons butter or margarine, melted
1   tablespoon finely chopped onion
    Salt and pepper to taste

Preheat oven to 325°F. Grease baking dish or casserole large enough to hold peppers standing up; set aside. Cut tops from peppers and remove seeds. In large saucepan or Dutch oven over medium heat, place peppers and ½ cup water. Cover and cook 5 minutes. Drain well upside down.

In medium bowl, combine remaining ingredients until thoroughly blended. Place peppers cut end up; fill evenly with corn mixture. Add 3 tablespoons water to dish. Bake about 1 hour, or until stuffing is set. Makes 4 servings.

Per serving: 143 calories; 6 g. protein; 6 g. fat; 38% calories from fat; 15 mg. cholesterol; 18 g. carbohydrates; 211 mg. sodium; 3 g. fiber

Spinach, Mushroom and Cheese Squares

2	pounds fresh spinach, trimmed
3	tablespoons butter or margarine
12	ounces fresh mushrooms, sliced
	Cholesterol-free, fat-free egg substitute, equivalent to 8 eggs
1½	cups soft whole-wheat bread crumbs
1¾	teaspoons salt
2	tablespoons Worcestershire sauce
2	cups low-fat cottage cheese

Preheat oven to 350°F. Grease 11 x 7-inch baking pan. Rinse spinach; drain or spin until almost dry. In large saucepot over medium heat, place damp spinach. Cover tightly and cook 2 to 3 minutes, or until just limp. Drain well and squeeze dry.

Heat butter or margarine in large skillet over medium heat. Sauté mushrooms 3 minutes, or until tender. In large bowl, combine spinach, ⅔ cooked mushrooms, egg substitute equivalent to 6 eggs, bread crumbs, 1 teaspoon salt and 1 tablespoon Worcestershire sauce until well blended. In medium bowl, combine remaining egg substitute, remaining 1 tablespoon Worcestershire sauce, remaining ¾ teaspoon salt and cottage cheese until well blended.

Into prepared baking pan, spoon ½ spinach mixture; top with all of cheese mixture, then remaining spinach mixture. Bake, uncovered, 30 minutes, or until firm. Let stand 10 minutes. Top with heated reserved mushrooms. Makes 6 servings.

Per serving: 225 calories; 25 g. protein; 8 g. fat; 30% calories from fat; 25 mg. cholesterol; 17 g. carbohydrates; 1345 mg. sodium; 8 g. fiber

Italian Stuffed Mushrooms

3   pounds large fresh mushrooms
2   medium onions, chopped
1-2 cloves garlic, minced
2   tablespoons dry sherry or white wine
1   tablespoon olive or other vegetable oil
1   package (10 ounces) frozen chopped spinach, thawed
    and squeezed dry
3   tablespoons Italian-seasoned dry bread crumbs
    Pinch dried oregano
    Pinch dried nutmeg
    Salt and pepper to taste
2   tablespoons grated sharp Romano or Parmesan cheese

Preheat oven to 375°F. Spray jelly-roll pan with nonstick cooking spray; set aside. Remove and finely chop stems from mushrooms. Reserve caps.

Spray large nonstick skillet with nonstick cooking spray; place over high heat. Add chopped mushrooms, onions, garlic, sherry or wine and oil; cook until liquid evaporates and mixture begins to lightly brown. Add spinach; cook until heated through. Remove from heat; stir in bread crumbs, oregano, nutmeg, salt and pepper until well mixed. On prepared pan, place mushroom caps top-side down; fill evenly with spinach mixture. Sprinkle with cheese. Bake 12 to 15 minutes, or until heated through. Makes 8 servings.

Per serving: 95 calories; 6 g. protein; 3 g. fat; 25% calories from fat; 1 mg. cholesterol; 14 g. carbohydrates; 78 mg. sodium; 5 g. fiber

Southern Pickled Shrimp

½ cup chopped celery leaves
¼ cup whole mixed pickling spice
1½ pounds frozen raw, peeled, deveined shrimp, thawed
2 cups sliced onions
5 bay leaves
1½ cups salad oil
1½ cups white vinegar
¼ cup chopped pimientos
2 tablespoons capers, undrained
1½ teaspoons celery seed
1½ teaspoons salt
¼ teaspoon hot-pepper sauce
    Salad greens for garnish (optional)

In small piece of cheesecloth, place celery and pickling spice; tie securely. In large saucepot or Dutch oven over high heat, bring to boil 2 quarts water and spice bag; boil 10 minutes. Add shrimp. Reduce heat to low; cover and simmer 3 to 5 minutes, or until shrimp are cooked. Drain.

In large bowl, arrange in layers onions and shrimp. Add bay leaves. In medium bowl, combine oil, vinegar, pimientos, capers, celery seed, salt and hot-pepper sauce until well mixed; pour over shrimp mixture. Cover and chill 6 hours, stirring occasionally. Drain well. To serve, place on bed of greens, if desired. Makes 6 servings.

Per serving: 193 calories; 24 g. protein; 8 g. fat; 39% calories from fat; 221 mg. cholesterol; 4 g. carbohydrates; 975 mg. sodium; 1 g. fiber

Broccoli Casserole

1   package (10 ounces) frozen chopped broccoli
1¼   cups lukewarm skim milk
     Cholesterol-free, fat-free egg substitute, equivalent to
      3 eggs
½   cup grated Parmesan or Romano cheese
½   teaspoon salt
½   teaspoon ground nutmeg

Preheat oven to 350°F. Grease 1½- to 2-quart casserole; set aside. Cook broccoli according to package directions; drain.

In small bowl, combine remaining ingredients; beat until well blended. Pour into prepared casserole. Add broccoli. Bake 25 to 30 minutes, or until knife inserted into center comes out clean. Serve immediately. Makes 4 servings.

Per serving: 115 calories; 13 g. protein; 3 g. fat; 25% calories from fat; 9 mg. cholesterol; 8 g. carbohydrates; 586 mg. sodium; 2 g. fiber

Spinach-Stuffed Tomatoes

6 medium firm, ripe tomatoes
  Salt
1 pound fresh, trimmed, chopped spinach, or 2 packages
  (10 ounces each) frozen chopped spinach, thawed
1 hard-cooked egg, finely chopped
1 tablespoon vinegar
½ teaspoon dried basil or tarragon (or ¼ teaspoon each)
¼ teaspoon dried oregano
⅛ teaspoon dried mustard
⅛ teaspoon garlic powder
¼ cup buttered bread crumbs*

Preheat oven to 350°F. Grease shallow casserole large enough to hold tomatoes; set aside. Cut tops off tomatoes; scoop out and reserve pulp, leaving ½-inch shells. Sprinkle shells with salt; invert to drain. Chop pulp. In small saucepan over low heat, place chopped tomato pulp, spinach and ¼ cup water; cook 5 minutes, stirring occasionally. Drain.

In medium bowl, combine tomato-spinach mixture, egg, vinegar, basil or tarragon, oregano, mustard and garlic powder until well blended. Place tomatoes cut end up in prepared casserole; fill with tomato-spinach mixture. Sprinkle tops with bread crumbs. Bake 20 minutes, or until tomato pierces easily with fork. Makes 3 servings.

Recipe for buttered bread crumbs is on page 154.
Per serving: 171 calories; 11 g. protein; 4 g. fat; 21% calories from fat; 95 mg. cholesterol; 27 g. carbohydrates; 277 mg. sodium; 9 g. fiber

Eggplant Italiano

2   medium eggplants (about 1 pound each), peeled and cut into 1-inch cubes

3   tablespoons olive or other vegetable oil

1   medium onion, finely chopped

2   cloves garlic, minced

⅓   cup finely chopped fresh parsley

2   medium green peppers, finely chopped

1   can (28 ounces) Italian-style tomatoes, broken up

3   tablespoons tomato paste

1½   teaspoons salt

1   teaspoon dried basil

½-1   teaspoon dried oregano

¼   teaspoon ground coriander

½   teaspoon pepper

3   tablespoons catsup

3   tablespoons chili sauce

    Salad greens, lemon slices, carrot curls, cherry tomatoes, black olives for garnish (optional)

Preheat oven to 350°F. Grease large baking pan; add eggplant cubes. Bake 45 minutes, or until soft, stirring frequently.

Heat oil in large heavy saucepan over medium heat. Sauté onions, garlic and parsley 5 to 7 minutes, or until soft. Add peppers; cook 3 minutes. Add tomatoes, tomato paste, salt, basil, oregano, coriander and pepper, mixing well. Reduce heat to low; cover and cook 20 to 30 minutes, stirring frequently.

In food processor or by hand, finely chop eggplant; add to tomato mixture. Cover and cook 20 minutes. Stir in catsup and chili sauce until well blended. Cover and chill several hours.

Serve on bed of greens with lemon slices and vegetable garnish, if desired. Makes 4 servings.

Per serving: 248 calories; 6 g. protein; 11 g. fat; 37% calories from fat; 0 mg. cholesterol; 36 g. carbohydrates; 1447 mg. sodium; 12 g. fiber

Ratatouille (Mixed Vegetables)

4   tablespoons canola, corn, cottonseed, safflower or soybean oil
3   large onions, finely chopped
3   large green peppers, coarsely chopped
6   small zucchini, thinly sliced
1   medium eggplant, unpeeled and cut into 1-inch cubes
6   large tomatoes, peeled, seeded and coarsely chopped
1   cup chopped fresh parsley
3   cloves garlic, minced
    Salt and pepper to taste
    Grated Parmesan cheese (optional)

Heat oil in large heavy skillet over medium heat. Sauté onions 5 minutes, or until light golden brown. Add peppers; cook 2 minutes. Stir in zucchini and eggplant; cook 5 minutes. Add tomatoes, parsley, garlic, salt and pepper, stirring until well mixed. Reduce heat to low; cook, covered, 15 to 20 minutes. Serve sprinkled with cheese, if desired.

Per serving: 258 calories; 5 g. protein; 15 g. fat; 49% calories from fat; 0 mg. cholesterol; 30 g. carbohydrates; 32 mg. sodium; 9 g. fiber

Eggplant Creole

1   medium eggplant, peeled and cut into 1-inch cubes
1¼   teaspoons salt
4   tablespoons butter or margarine
3   tablespoons all-purpose flour
3   large tomatoes, peeled and chopped
1   small green pepper, chopped
1   small onion, chopped
1   tablespoon brown sugar
2   whole cloves
1   small bay leaf
¼   cup dry bread crumbs

Preheat oven to 350°F. Grease 1½-quart casserole; set aside. In medium saucepan over medium heat, cook eggplant, ¾ teaspoon salt and ½ cup water, uncovered, 10 minutes, or until eggplant is tender. Drain well; place in prepared casserole.

Melt 3 tablespoons butter or margarine in large skillet over medium heat. Stir in flour until blended. Add remaining ½ teaspoon salt, tomatoes, peppers, onions, brown sugar, cloves and bay leaf. Cook, uncovered, 5 minutes, stirring occasionally. Remove bay leaf; pour mixture over eggplant. Sprinkle with bread crumbs; dot with remaining tablespoon butter or margarine. Bake 30 minutes. Makes 4 servings.

Per serving: 199 calories; 3 g. protein; 12 g. fat; 51% calories from fat; 31 mg. cholesterol; 22 g. carbohydrates; 780 mg. sodium; 6 g. fiber

Stuffed Squash

2   acorn squash
2   cups chopped mushrooms
1   cup chopped onions
2   cloves garlic, crushed
2   tablespoons dry white wine
¼   cup chopped parsley
1   teaspoon tamari or lite soy sauce
½   teaspoon dried basil or thyme
     Pepper to taste
1   cup low-fat cottage cheese
¾   cup cooked brown rice or bread crumbs

Preheat oven to 350°F. Pierce squash with fork; bake in oven or microwave until tender. Cut in half and remove seeds; set aside. In large skillet over medium heat, cook mushrooms, onions, garlic and wine 3 minutes, or until onions are tender. Add parsley, tamari or soy sauce, basil or thyme and pepper; cook 1 minute. Remove from heat; stir in cottage cheese and rice or bread crumbs until well blended. Let stand 2 minutes; drain, reserving liquid for sauce.

In large casserole, place acorn squash; fill with vegetable-cheese mixture. Bake for 30 minutes, or until heated through. In small saucepan, cook drained liquid until of desired sauce consistency, stirring occasionally. Serve over squash. Makes 4 servings.

Per serving: 235 calories; 11 g. protein; 1 g. fat; 5% calories from fat; 7 mg. cholesterol; 49 g. carbohydrates; 289 mg. sodium; 8 g. fiber

Spicy Yellow Squash

2 tablespoons butter or margarine
8 medium yellow summer squash, sliced 1-inch thick
1 medium onion, finely chopped
2 hot chili peppers, stems and seeds removed
2 medium tomatoes, peeled and chopped
½ cup diced ham
  Salt and pepper to taste
¼ cup shredded reduced-fat Cheddar cheese

Preheat oven to 350°F. Grease 2- to 2½-quart casserole; set aside. Melt butter or margarine in large skillet over medium heat. Sauté squash, onions and chili peppers 3 minutes, or until onions are tender. Add tomatoes, ham, salt and pepper. Cook, stirring, 1 minute; pour into prepared casserole. Sprinkle with cheese. Bake 10 to 15 minutes, or until cheese melts and browns slightly. Makes 4 servings.

Note: If desired, ½ large green pepper, chopped, may be substituted for chili peppers.

Per serving: 170 calories; 10 g. protein; 8 g. fat; 42% calories from fat; 27 mg. cholesterol; 16 g. carbohydrates; 343 mg. sodium; 5 g. fiber

Vegetable Casserole

4 medium potatoes (about 1¼ pounds), peeled and
     thinly sliced
   Salt and pepper to taste
4 tablespoons butter or margarine, cut into pieces
2 medium onions, thinly sliced and separated into rings
4 small yellow summer squash (about 1¼ pounds),
     thinly sliced
1 cup nonfat sour cream
½ cup grated Parmesan cheese

Preheat oven to 350°F. Grease 2½-quart ovenproof and broilerproof casserole; layer ½ potatoes, salt, pepper and ½ tablespoon butter or margarine; ½ onions, salt, pepper and ½ tablespoon butter or margarine; and ½ squash, salt, pepper and 1 tablespoon butter. Repeat layers.

Cover tightly; bake 1 to 1¼ hours, or until potatoes are fork-tender. In small bowl, stir sour cream and cheese until well blended; spoon over casserole. Broil until lightly browned. To serve, spoon down through all layers. Makes 6 servings.

Per serving: 260 calories; 7 g. protein; 10 g. fat; 35% calories from fat; 32 mg. cholesterol; 34 g. carbohydrates; 252 mg. sodium; 3 g. fiber

Baked Zucchini and Rice Soufflé

3   medium zucchini (about 1 pound), thickly sliced
½   cup cooked rice
6   ounces nonfat sour cream
1   cup (4 ounces) shredded Swiss cheese
    Cholesterol-free, fat-free egg substitute, equivalent to
      2 eggs
    Salt and pepper to taste

Preheat oven to 350°F. Grease 1-quart casserole; set aside. In medium saucepan over medium heat, cook zucchini in lightly salted water 7 to 10 minutes, or until tender. Drain well; place into prepared casserole. Top with rice. In small bowl, stir sour cream, cheese, egg substitute, salt and pepper until well blended; pour over rice. Bake for 40 minutes, or until brown. Makes 4 servings.

Per serving: 202 calories; 14 g. protein; 8 g. fat; 37% calories from fat; 32 mg. cholesterol; 16 g. carbohydrates; 181 mg. sodium; 1 g. fiber

Potato and Spinach Casserole

3   medium potatoes (about 1 pound), peeled and cut
     into eighths
2   eggs, at room temperature, separated
4   tablespoons butter or margarine
½   teaspoon white pepper or to taste
¼   teaspoon ground nutmeg or to taste
1½ bags (10 ounces each) fresh spinach, trimmed
3   tablespoons grated Parmesan cheese
     Parsley sprigs for garnish (optional)

Preheat oven to 400°F. Grease 2-quart casserole; set aside. In medium saucepan over medium-high heat, place potatoes and ½ cup lightly salted water. Cover and cook 20 minutes, or until fork-tender; drain. Mash or put through potato ricer. Add egg yolks, 1½ tablespoons butter or margarine, pepper and nutmeg, stirring until almost smooth. In small bowl with mixer, beat egg whites until stiff peaks form; fold into potato mixture and set aside.

Rinse spinach; drain or spin almost dry. In large saucepot over medium heat, place damp spinach. Cover tightly and cook 2 to 3 minutes, or until just limp. Drain well; add 1½ tablespoons butter or margarine; toss until well coated.

Spoon ½ potato mixture into prepared casserole; top with spinach mixture, then remaining potato mixture. Sprinkle with cheese and dot with remaining 1 tablespoon butter or margarine. Bake 30 minutes, or until heated through. Garnish with parsley, if desired. Makes 4 servings.

Per serving: 263 calories; 8 g. protein; 14 g. fat; 49% calories from fat; 168 mg. cholesterol; 27 g. carbohydrates; 226 mg. sodium; 5 g. fiber

Spinach Pie

2   packages (10 ounces each) frozen chopped spinach,
      cooked and drained
     Cholesterol-free, fat-free egg substitute, equivalent to
      2 eggs
1   cup (4 ounces) shredded Swiss cheese
1   unbaked 9-inch pie crust
1   cup nonfat sour cream
1   tablespoon butter or margarine
4   tablespoons Italian-seasoned dry bread crumbs

Preheat oven to 350°F. In medium bowl, combine spinach, egg substitute and cheese; spoon into pie crust. Cover top completely with layer of sour cream. Melt butter or margarine in small skillet. Cook bread crumbs, stirring, until lightly browned; sprinkle over top. Bake 45 minutes, or until knife comes out clean. Makes 8 servings.

Per serving: 195 calories; 6 g. protein; 9 g. fat; 43% calories from fat; 9 mg. cholesterol; 21 g. carbohydrates; 298 mg. sodium; 2 g. fiber

Broccoli-Mushroom Stir-Fry

2   tablespoons corn oil
¾   pound broccoli, trimmed and cut into florets, with
    stems sliced
1¼ cups sliced mushrooms
1   large carrot, cut into 2-inch strips
1   clove garlic, minced
1   teaspoon shredded lemon peel
½   teaspoon salt
¼   teaspoon dried thyme

Heat oil in large skillet or wok over medium-high heat. Add remaining ingredients. Cook, stirring constantly, 5 to 8 minutes, or until vegetables are tender. Makes 4 servings.

Per serving: 97 calories; 3 g. protein; 7 g. fat; 61% calories from fat; 0 mg. cholesterol; 7 g. carbohydrates; 297 mg. sodium; 3 g. fiber

Cauliflower-Pasta Toss

3   cups uncooked penne, rigatoni or ziti
2   tablespoons butter or margarine
2   tablespoons olive oil
1   clove garlic, minced
1   package (10 ounces) frozen cauliflower, cooked
¼   teaspoon dried oregano
½   tablespoon dehydrated parsley flakes
    Salt and pepper to taste
    Grated Parmesan cheese (optional)

Prepare pasta according to package directions. Heat butter or margarine and oil in large skillet over medium heat. Sauté garlic 2 minutes. Add cauliflower; sauté 5 minutes, or until lightly browned. Drain pasta; add to cauliflower with oregano, parsley, salt and pepper. Heat through. Serve sprinkled with cheese, if desired. Makes 4 servings.

Per serving: 517 calories; 14 g. protein; 14 g. fat; 24% calories from fat; 15 mg. cholesterol; 82 g. carbohydrates; 63 mg. sodium; 6 g. fiber

Asparagus-Tomato Stir-Fry

1   tablespoon cold water
2   teaspoons soy sauce
1   teaspoon cornstarch
¼   teaspoon salt
1   tablespoon corn or blended vegetable oil
1   pound fresh asparagus, diagonally sliced into 1-inch
      pieces
4   green onions with tops, diagonally sliced into 1-inch
      pieces
½   cup sliced fresh mushrooms
2   small tomatoes, cut into thin wedges

In small bowl or custard cup, stir water, soy sauce, cornstarch and salt until thoroughly blended; set aside. Heat oil in large skillet or wok over medium-high heat. Add asparagus and onions. Cook, stirring constantly, 4 minutes. Add mushrooms; cook, stirring constantly, 2 minutes more. Push vegetables to side; stir cornstarch mixture and add to skillet or wok. Cook, stirring into vegetables, until sauce thickens and bubbles. Add tomatoes. Toss gently to combine. Serve immediately. Makes 6 servings.

Per serving: 49 calories; 3 g. protein; 2 g. fat; 40% calories from fat; 0 mg. cholesterol; 5 g. carbohydrates; 208 mg. sodium; 2 g. fiber

Bulgur-Cheese Stuffed Peppers

6   large green peppers
3   tablespoons olive oil
1   small onion, finely chopped
1   large carrot, shredded
½   teaspoon dried basil
½   teaspoon dried oregano
2   cloves garlic, minced
2½ cups cooked bulgur (cracked wheat)
1½ cups (6 ounces) shredded part-skim milk mozzarella
    cheese
2   eggs, beaten
    Salt and pepper to taste
1   cup tomato juice

Preheat oven to 350°F. Grease baking dish or casserole large enough to hold peppers standing up; set aside. Cut tops from peppers and remove seeds. In large saucepan or Dutch oven over medium heat, place peppers and ½ cup water. Cover and cook 5 minutes. Drain well upside down.

Heat oil in small skillet over medium heat. Sauté onions and carrots 3 minutes, or until tender. Add basil, oregano and garlic. In large bowl, stir onion-carrot mixture, bulgur, cheese, eggs, salt and pepper. In prepared dish, place peppers cut end up; fill evenly with bulgur mixture. Add tomato juice to dish. Cover and bake 20 to 25 minutes, or until stuffing is set. Makes 6 servings.

Per serving: 306 calories; 15 g. protein; 14 g. fat; 43% calories from fat; 43 mg. cholesterol; 28 g. carbohydrates; 328 mg. sodium; 6 g. fiber

Green and Yellow Pasta

8 ounces spinach pasta
8 ounces regular pasta
2 tablespoons butter or margarine
3 cups cubed zucchini
2 cloves garlic, minced
2 cups nonfat plain yogurt
3 tablespoons chopped fresh basil or parsley
   Grated Parmesan cheese (optional)

Cook pasta al dente according to package directions. Melt butter or margarine in large skillet over medium heat. Sauté zucchini and garlic until golden. Turn off heat; stir in yogurt and basil or parsley. Drain pasta; toss immediately with yogurt mixture. Serve with cheese, if desired. Makes 4 servings.

Note: For slightly thicker, richer sauce, 1 cup each nonfat plain yogurt and nonfat sour cream may be used instead of all yogurt.

Per serving: 294 calories; 13 g. protein; 6 g. fat; 20% calories from fat; 17 mg. cholesterol; 45 g. carbohydrates; 138 mg. sodium; 3 g. fiber

All Green and White Sandwich

4 large (7- to 8-inch) pita breads (Middle Eastern pocket bread)
1 small zucchini, thinly sliced
1 small green pepper, chopped
4 green onions, chopped
1 cup bean sprouts or alfalfa sprouts
1 cup coarsely chopped spinach leaves
4 ounces feta cheese, crumbled
4 ounces nonfat plain yogurt

Slice off top inch of pita breads. Holding bread open, drop cut-off portion into bottom. In small bowl, combine zucchini, peppers, green onions, sprouts, spinach, and cheese. Place ¼ vegetable mixture in each pita. Stir yogurt until thinned down; pour ¼ over vegetable mixture in each pita. Makes 4 servings.

Per serving: 278 calories; 14 g. protein; 7 g. fat; 23% calories from fat; 25 mg. cholesterol; 40 g. carbohydrates; 690 mg. sodium; 3 g. fiber

Kidney Bean and Corn Chili

2	tablespoons canola, corn, cottonseed, safflower or soybean oil
1	small onion, chopped
1	clove garlic, minced
½	cup chopped green peppers
2	cups thawed frozen or drained canned whole-kernel corn
1	cup water
1½	tablespoons tomato paste
3	cups cooked or drained canned kidney beans
1	teaspoon dried oregano
½-1	teaspoon chili powder
¼	teaspoon ground cumin

Heat oil in large skillet over medium heat. Sauté onions and garlic 3 minutes. Add peppers; cook 3 minutes. Add corn, water and tomato paste. In small bowl with fork, mash 1 cup beans. Add mashed beans, remaining 2 cups whole beans, oregano, chili powder and cumin to skillet mixture. Bring to boil. Reduce heat to low; simmer 30 minutes, or until thickened. Makes 4 servings.

Per serving: 311 calories; 14 g. protein; 7 g. fat; 21% calories from fat; 0 mg. cholesterol; 50 g. carbohydrates; 12 mg. sodium; 15 g. fiber

Vegetable Loaf

1   large carrot
1   rib celery
½   cup chopped broccoli
2   ounces green beans, cooked
1   tablespoon safflower oil
1   small onion, chopped
1   cup soft bread crumbs
1   egg
     Salt and pepper to taste
¼   teaspoon nutmeg or ground ginger

Preheat oven to 350°F. Grease shallow baking dish; set aside. Through grinder or in food processor, coarsely grind or chop carrot, celery, broccoli and green beans. Heat oil in large skillet over medium heat. Sauté onions 3 minutes or until tender. Add to chopped vegetables with remaining ingredients; shape into loaf. Place in prepared dish. Bake 45 minutes, or until firm. Makes 4 servings.

Per serving: 107 calories; 4 g. protein; 5 g. fat; 44% calories from fat; 68 mg. cholesterol; 11 g. carbohydrates; 92 mg. sodium; 2 g. fiber

Vegetable Stew

2   potatoes, peeled and cubed
2   carrots, peeled and sliced
2   ribs celery, cut into slices
2   medium onions, sliced
1   large red pepper, cut into strips
1   clove garlic, minced
½   head broccoflower, cut into florets
½   pound mushrooms, sliced
1   can (13¾ ounces) ready-to-use chicken broth
2   tablespoons chopped fresh dill, or 2 teaspoons
       dried dill
2   teaspoons salt
⅛   teaspoon pepper

Preheat oven to 350°F. Place all ingredients in 3-quart casserole. Cover and bake 45 to 60 minutes, or until vegetables are of desired doneness. Makes 8 servings.

Per serving: 88 calories; 4 g. protein; 0 g. fat; 7% calories from fat; 0 mg. cholesterol, 18 g. carbohydrates; 723 mg. sodium; 4 g. fiber

Lentil Burgers

2   cups cooked lentils*
2   eggs, lightly beaten
1   cup soft whole-wheat bread crumbs
½   cup wheat germ
½   cup finely chopped onions
1¼ teaspoons salt
    Dash hot-pepper sauce
2   tablespoons canola, corn, cottonseed, safflower or
    soybean oil
    Whole-wheat hamburger rolls or pita breads (optional)

In medium bowl, mash lentils slightly. Add eggs, bread crumbs, wheat germ, onions, salt and hot-pepper sauce. Shape ½-cup portions lentil mixture into six 3 ½-inch patties. Heat oil in large skillet over medium heat. Fry patties, turning once, 5 minutes, or until golden brown. Serve in rolls or pitas, if desired. Makes 6 servings.

About ¾ cup uncooked lentils equals 2 cups cooked.

Per serving: 204 calories; 11 g. protein; 10 g. fat; 34% calories from fat; 91 mg. cholesterol; 22 g. carbohydrates; 508 mg. sodium; 5 g. fiber

Chicken à la King

⅓ cup water
1 cup frozen green peas
¼ cup chopped green peppers
2 tablespoons finely chopped onions
⅔ cup all-purpose flour
1 cup cold skim milk
2 cups chicken broth or bouillon
2 teaspoons salt
½ teaspoon poultry seasoning
   Pepper to taste
2 cups diced cooked chicken or turkey
1 can (4 ounces) mushroom stems and pieces, drained
   and coarsely chopped
1 tablespoon chopped pimientos
   Toast, biscuits or cooked rice (optional)

In medium saucepan over medium heat, place water, peas, peppers and onions. Cover and cook 5 minutes, or until peas are tender. Drain, saving liquid.

In same saucepan, blend flour and milk until well blended; stir in reserved cooking liquid, broth or bouillon, salt, poultry seasoning and pepper. Bring to boil, stirring constantly. Cook 1 minute. Add cooked vegetables, chicken or turkey, mushrooms and pimientos. Heat through. Serve over rice, toast or biscuits, if desired. Makes 6 servings.

Per serving: 178 calories; 17 g. protein; 3 g. fat; 18% calories from fat; 39 mg. cholesterol; 18 g. carbohydrates; 1113 mg. sodium; 2 g. fiber

Mushroom and Chicken Kabobs

1   can (8 ounces) pineapple chunks in juice
2   tablespoons canola, corn, cottonseed, safflower or
      soybean oil
¾   teaspoon garlic powder
¾   teaspoon ground ginger
¼   teaspoon salt
1½ pounds boneless, skinless chicken breasts,
      cut into 1½-inch chunks
1   pound fresh mushrooms, cut in half
1   large green pepper, cut into chunks
      Hot cooked rice (optional)

Drain pineapple, reserving juice; set chunks aside. In small bowl, combine reserved juice, oil, garlic powder, ginger and salt until well mixed. In large bowl, place chicken; pour in oil mixture and toss to coat evenly. Cover and chill for 2 hours, stirring occasionally.

Preheat broiler. Assemble 12 7-inch skewers. Drain chicken, reserving marinade. Thread each skewer with mushroom half, pepper chunk and chicken chunk; repeat. Place pineapple chunk on end. Place any remaining pineapple chunks on skewers. Brush skewers with reserved marinade. Broil 6 inches from heat source, turning frequently, 5 minutes, or until chicken is tender. Serve over rice, if desired. Makes 6 servings.

Per serving: 209 calories; 28 g. protein; 6 g. fat; 27% calories from fat; 65 mg. cholesterol; 10 g. carbohydrates; 166 mg. sodium; 2 g. fiber

Curried Chicken with Rice

2½   pounds whole chicken breasts, split
1   teaspoon salt
3   tablespoons canola, corn, cottonseed, safflower or
     soybean oil
1   cup green pepper strips
¼   pound fresh mushrooms, sliced
½   cup chopped onions
1   clove garlic, minced
2   cans (10½ ounces each) condensed chicken broth
1½   cups uncooked long-grain rice
1   teaspoon curry powder
1   package (6 ounces) frozen snow pea pods, thawed
1   medium tomato, chopped

Sprinkle chicken with ¾ teaspoon salt. Heat oil in large skillet over medium-high heat. Add chicken; cook 7 minutes, or until brown on both sides. Push to one side of skillet. Add peppers, mushrooms, onions and garlic; sauté 5 minutes or until onions are tender.

In 4-cup measure, add enough water to chicken broth to make 3¼ cups. To chicken-vegetable mixture, add diluted broth, remaining ¼ teaspoon salt, rice and curry powder. Rearrange chicken breasts on top of rice mixture. Bring to boil. Reduce heat to low; cover and simmer, stirring occasionally, for 15 minutes, or until chicken is tender. Add pea pods and tomatoes. Cover and cook for 2 minutes, or until rice is tender and liquid is absorbed. Serve immediately. Makes 6 servings.

Per serving: 426 calories; 39 g. protein; 9 g. fat; 20% calories from fat; 82 mg. cholesterol; 43 g. carbohydrates; 944 mg. sodium; 3 g. fiber

Chicken Cacciatore

¼   cup all-purpose flour
1   teaspoon salt
¼   teaspoon pepper
1   broiler-fryer chicken (about 2½ pounds), cut into
      pieces and skinned
3   tablespoons olive or other vegetable oil
½   cup drained canned small white pearl onions, or
      thawed frozen small white pearl onions
1   medium green pepper, cut into strips
1   can (4 ounces) mushrooms, drained
1   clove garlic, minced
½   cup water
1   can (10½ ounces) condensed tomato soup
2   tablespoons vinegar or lemon juice
1   tablespoon Worcestershire sauce
½   teaspoon dried oregano
      Hot cooked spaghetti (optional)

On wax paper, mix flour, salt and pepper. Roll chicken into flour mixture until well coated. Heat oil in large skillet over medium heat. Cook chicken 7 minutes, or until brown on both sides; remove and keep warm. To same skillet, add onions, peppers, mushrooms and garlic; sauté 5 minutes, or until tender.

In small bowl, combine water, undiluted tomato soup, vinegar or lemon juice, Worcestershire sauce and oregano until well blended; pour into skillet. Add chicken; cover and simmer, stirring occasionally, about 30 minutes, or until chicken is fork-tender. Serve over spaghetti, if desired. Makes 4 servings.

Per serving: 412 calories; 40 g. protein; 16 g. fat; 36% calories from fat; 119 mg. cholesterol; 26 g. carbohydrates; 1577 mg. sodium; 2 g. fiber

Tomatoes Stuffed with Chicken

1	cup nonfat plain yogurt
½	teaspoon salt
¼	teaspoon tarragon
1½	cups diced cooked chicken
1	can (8 ounces) crushed pineapple, drained
3	tablespoons toasted slivered almonds
1	rib celery, finely chopped
6	large tomatoes

In small bowl, combine yogurt, salt and tarragon; set aside. In large bowl, combine chicken, pineapple, almonds and celery. Add yogurt mixture; toss gently to evenly coat. To serve, cut tomatoes into wedges almost to bottom; gently spread out. Fill each with ⅙ chicken mixture. Makes 6 servings.

Per serving: 151 calories; 14 g. protein; 5 g. fat; 30% calories from fat; 32 mg. cholesterol; 13 g. carbohydrates; 253 mg. sodium; 3 g. fiber

Poule au Pot

  1   stewing or roasting chicken (about 5 pounds)
 16   cups water
 12   small pearl onions, peeled
  6   ribs celery, cut into 2-inch lengths
  4   small turnips, peeled and quartered (2 cups)
  3   medium carrots, cut into 2-inch lengths
  2   green peppers, cored, seeded and cut into quarters
 1½   cups chopped leeks
  2   bay leaves
  2   cloves garlic, peeled and left whole
 12   peppercorns
 1½   teaspoons dried thyme
      Salt and pepper to taste
  3   small zucchini, cut into 1-inch lengths
  2   medium parsnips, peeled and cut into quarters
  ⅔   cup uncooked rice

In large Dutch oven over high heat, place chicken, water, onions, celery, turnips, carrots, green peppers, leeks, bay leaves, garlic, peppercorns, thyme, salt and pepper. Bring to boil. Reduce heat to low; cover and cook 45 to 75 minutes, or until chicken is almost tender. Add remaining ingredients; cook 15 minutes, or until rice is tender. Remove bay leaves; skin chicken. Makes 8 servings.

Per serving: 511 calories; 58 g. protein; 14 g. fat; 25% calories from fat; 164 mg. cholesterol; 35 g. carbohydrates; 207 mg. sodium; 7 g. fiber

Moo Goo Gai Pan (Chicken with Pea Pods)

1   pound boneless, skinless chicken, cut into strips
3   tablespoons soy sauce
4   ribs celery, cut into 1-inch strips
2   medium onions, sliced
1   can (16 ounces) mixed Chinese vegetables, drained
1   can (4 ounces) mushrooms, drained
¾   cup hot water
2   chicken bouillon cubes
2   tablespoons cornstarch
1   package (6 ounces) frozen snow pea pods
     Hot cooked rice (optional)

In large skillet over medium heat, place chicken and 2 tablespoons soy sauce. Cook, stirring, 5 minutes, or until chicken is no longer pink; remove. To skillet, add celery, onions, Chinese vegetables and mushrooms. In 1-cup measure, combine water, remaining tablespoon soy sauce and bouillon cubes, stirring until bouillon is dissolved. Add to vegetables; cook 15 minutes. Add chicken; cook 5 minutes. In small bowl, blend 2 tablespoons cold water and cornstarch until well mixed. Add to skillet with pea pods; cook, stirring occasionally, 3 minutes, or until thickened. Makes 4 servings.

Per serving: 254 calories; 33 g. protein; 2 g. fat; 8% calories from fat; 65 mg. cholesterol; 26 g. carbohydrates; 1392 mg. sodium; 7 g. fiber

Braised Chicken and Vegetables

5   tablespoons all-purpose flour
    Salt and pepper to taste
1   broiler-fryer chicken (about 2½ pounds), cut up
2   tablespoons corn oil
3   medium carrots, cut up
½   pound mushrooms, sliced
4   ribs celery, chopped
½   large onion, chopped
½   large green pepper, chopped
1½   cups water

On wax paper, mix well 3 tablespoons flour, salt and pepper. Roll chicken into flour mixture until well coated. Heat oil in large saucepot or Dutch oven over medium heat. Cook chicken 7 minutes, or until brown on both sides; remove and keep warm. To same saucepot, add remaining flour and remaining ingredients. Bring to boil. Add reserved chicken. Reduce heat to low; cover and cook 45 minutes, or until chicken is tender. Makes 4 servings.

Per serving: 375 calories; 45 g. protein; 12 g. fat; 30% calories from fat; 139 mg. cholesterol; 18 g. carbohydrates; 206 mg. sodium; 4 g. fiber

Hawaiian Chicken

1 broiler-fryer chicken (about 2½ pounds), cut up
   Salt and pepper to taste
1¼ cups orange juice
½ cup prepared chutney
½ cup raisins
½ teaspoon ground cinnamon
½ teaspoon curry powder
½ teaspoon dried thyme
¼ cup blanched slivered almonds

Preheat oven to 425°F. Grease baking dish or roasting pan large enough to hold chicken in single layer; add chicken. Season with salt and pepper. Bake 15 minutes.

In medium saucepan over high heat, combine orange juice, chutney, raisins, cinnamon, curry powder and thyme; bring to boil. Pour over chicken. Bake 45 to 50 minutes more, or until chicken is fork-tender. Sprinkle with almonds last 5 minutes. Makes 4 servings.

Per serving: 383 calories; 45 g. protein; 9 g. fat; 23% calories from fat; 139 mg. cholesterol; 29 g. carbohydrates; 154 mg. sodium; 3 g. fiber

Turkey-Leek Rotini

1   package (16 ounces) rotini or other short pasta
3   tablespoons butter or margarine
1   pound leeks, white part and 2 inches of green stem
       quartered lengthwise and sliced
¼   cup all-purpose flour
    Salt and pepper to taste
1   pound boneless turkey breast fillets, cut into 1x1¼-
       inch slivers
2   tablespoons canola, corn, cottonseed, safflower or
       soybean oil
¼   cup white port, other dry white wine or chicken broth
¾   cup skim milk
½   cup (2 ounces) shredded Muenster cheese
¼   cup (1 ounce) blue cheese, crumbled
¼   cup chopped fresh Italian parsley

Cook pasta according to package directions. Meanwhile, melt 1 tablespoon butter or margarine in large skillet over medium-high heat. Sauté leeks, stirring often, 5 minutes, or until leeks are wilted. Remove leeks; keep warm.

On wax paper, combine flour, salt and pepper. Dip turkey into flour mixture to coat well. To same skillet, add remaining butter or margarine and oil. Add coated turkey in batches; cook, stirring, 5 minutes, or until golden. Remove; keep warm.

Add wine or broth to skillet over medium-high heat, scraping skillet bottom to remove browned bits. Cook 1 minute. Add reserved leeks, browned turkey, milk, cheeses and parsley. Drain pasta. On large platter, place pasta; top with sauce. Toss gently to evenly coat. Serve immediately. Makes 6 servings.

Per serving: 303 calories; 22 g. protein; 16 g. fat; 50% calories from fat; 67 mg. cholesterol; 13 g. carbohydrates; 238 mg. sodium; 1 g. fiber

Turkey and Rice Stuffed Peppers

4	large green peppers
2	cups ½-inch cubes cooked turkey
1	cup hot, cooked rice
¼	pound fresh mushrooms, chopped
1	jar (2 ounces) chopped pimientos, undrained
½	cup light mayonnaise
¼	cup nonfat sour cream
2	tablespoons instant chicken bouillon granules
1	tablespoon dried parsley
½	teaspoon celery salt
½	teaspoon hot pepper sauce
¼	teaspoon ground thyme

Preheat oven to 375°F. Grease baking dish or casserole large enough to hold peppers standing up. Cut tops from peppers and remove seeds. Place cut end up in prepared dish; set aside. In large bowl, combine remaining ingredients until well blended; fill peppers. Add 1 cup water to dish; cover tightly with lid or foil. Bake 45 to 50 minutes, or until peppers are tender-crisp. Makes 4 servings.

Per serving: 322 calories; 23 g. protein; 14 g. fat; 41% calories from fat; 66 mg. cholesterol; 23 g. carbohydrates; 587 mg. sodium; 2 g. fiber

Turkey Parmigiana

2   egg whites or cholesterol-free, fat-free egg substitute, equivalent to 2 eggs
2   tablespoons canola, cottonseed, corn, safflower or soybean oil
⅓   cup Italian-seasoned dry bread crumbs
½   teaspoon salt
     Dash pepper
1   pound raw turkey breast slices
¾   cup defatted turkey or chicken broth
3   tablespoons tomato paste
1   clove garlic, minced
1   teaspoon dried oregano
1   cup (4 ounces) part-skim milk mozzarella cheese

Preheat oven to 450°F. Spray jelly-roll pan with nonstick cooking spray; set aside. In shallow dish, beat eggs and oil until well blended. On wax paper, mix bread crumbs, salt and pepper. Dip each turkey slice into egg mixture, then into bread crumbs to lightly coat both sides. Arrange in single layer on prepared pan. Bake 8 to 10 minutes, or until golden and crisp. Place in single layer in ovenproof and broilerproof casserole or platter; keep warm.

Preheat broiler. In small saucepan over medium heat, combine broth, tomato paste, garlic and oregano. Cook, uncovered, until thickened to desired consistency. Spoon over turkey; top with cheese. Broil until cheese lightly browns. Makes 4 servings.

Per serving: 324 calories; 36 g. protein; 14 g. fat; 42% calories from fat; 75 mg. cholesterol; 10 g. carbohydrates; 825 mg. sodium; 1 g. fiber

Vegetable-Burger Potpourri

8 ounces ground chicken, turkey or beef
2 cups water
1 can (16 ounces) stewed tomatoes, cut up
1 can (8 ounces) tomato sauce
1 package (10 ounces) frozen mixed vegetables
½ envelope (¼ cup) dry onion soup mix
1 teaspoon sugar
   Dash Worcestershire sauce
   Dash garlic salt

In large heavy saucepan or Dutch oven over medium heat, cook chicken, turkey or beef, stirring occasionally, 5 minutes, or until browned; drain off excess fat. Stir in remaining ingredients. Bring to boil. Reduce heat to low; cover and simmer 20 minutes, or until vegetables are cooked. Makes 6 servings.

Per serving: 121 calories; 9 g. protein; 4 g. fat; 28% calories from fat; 35 mg. cholesterol; 13 g. carbohydrates; 450 mg. sodium; 3 g. fiber

Noodles Milanese

2 tablespoons canola, corn, cottonseed, safflower or
soybean oil
2 medium onions, chopped
1 clove garlic, minced
1 pound lean ground beef
1 can (8 ounces) tomato sauce
1 can (6 ounces) tomato paste
1 teaspoon dried oregano
Salt to taste
8 ounces uncooked noodles
2 eggs
¾ pound fresh spinach, trimmed, cooked,
and chopped, or 1 package (10 ounces)
frozen chopped spinach, thawed
1 cup low-fat cottage cheese
½ cup chopped fresh parsley
½ cup grated Parmesan cheese
1 teaspoon dried basil

Preheat oven to 350°F. Grease 12 x 8-inch baking dish; set
aside. Heat oil in large skillet over medium heat. Sauté onions
and garlic 3 minutes, or until tender. Add beef; cook, stirring,
5 minutes, or until brown. Add tomato sauce, tomato paste,
oregano and salt. Reduce heat to low; simmer 15 minutes.

Cook noodles according to package directions; drain. In
large bowl, stir drained noodles and 1 egg; set aside. In another
bowl, stir remaining egg, spinach, cottage cheese, parsley, ¼ cup
Parmesan cheese and basil until well blended. In prepared pan,
layer ½ noodle mixture, ⅓ tomato-beef mixture, and ½ spinach

mixture; repeat layers. Top with remaining tomato-beef mixture and ¼ cup Parmesan cheese. Bake 45 minutes, or until heated through. Let stand 5 minutes. Makes 6 servings.

Per serving: 526 calories; 35 g. protein; 27 g. fat; 46% calories from fat; 201 mg. cholesterol; 36 g. carbohydrates; 608 mg. sodium; 5 g. fiber

Carrot Meat Loaf

1	pound lean ground beef
2	large carrots, shredded (about 1½ cups)
1	medium onion, chopped
½	cup cornflake crumbs
½	cup skim milk
1	egg
1	teaspoon Worcestershire sauce
1	teaspoon salt
½	teaspoon pepper

Preheat oven to 350°F. In large bowl, combine all ingredients until well blended. Place in 8 x 4-inch loaf pan; bake 50 to 60 minutes, or until done. Drain off fat; let stand 10 minutes. Remove from pan and slice. Makes 6 servings.

Per serving: 261 calories; 21 g. protein; 15 g. fat; 53% calories from fat; 112 mg. cholesterol; 9 g. carbohydrates; 505 mg. sodium; 1 g. fiber

Little Joes

¾ pound fresh spinach, trimmed, or 1 bag (10 ounces) fresh spinach, trimmed

1 tablespoon canola, corn, cottonseed, safflower or soybean oil

1 cup finely chopped onions

1 pound lean ground beef

Salt and pepper to taste

Cholesterol-free, fat-free egg substitute, equivalent to 4 eggs

Hot-pepper sauce to taste

¼ cup grated Parmesan cheese

Rinse spinach; drain or spin dry. In large saucepot over medium heat, place damp spinach. Cover and cook 1 to 2 minutes, or until wilted. Cool and squeeze dry; chop and set aside. Heat oil in medium heavy skillet over medium heat. Sauté onions 3 minutes, or until tender. Add beef; cook, stirring, to brown and break up lumps. Add spinach, salt and pepper, stirring until blended. Pour eggs and hot-pepper sauce over meat-spinach mixture. Cook, gently stirring, until eggs are set. Top with cheese. Makes 6 servings.

Per serving: 284 calories; 26 g. protein; 17 g. fat; 56% calories from fat; 68 mg. cholesterol; 5 g. carbohydrates; 240 mg. sodium; 2 g. fiber

Fish Fillets on Spinach

1½ pounds boneless, skinless fish fillets (cod, turbot, flounder, orange roughy)
2 tablespoons lemon juice
1½ pounds fresh spinach, trimmed and chopped, or 2 bags (10 ounces each) frozen chopped spinach
1 tablespoon canola, cottonseed, corn, safflower or soybean oil
1 medium onion, chopped
½ teaspoon salt
½ teaspoon ground nutmeg
⅛ teaspoon white pepper
2 medium tomatoes, sliced
¼ cup (1 ounce) shredded part-skim milk mozzarella cheese

Preheat oven to 350°F. Grease shallow 2½-quart casserole; set aside. Sprinkle fish with lemon juice; let stand 10 minutes. Rinse spinach; drain or spin dry. Heat oil in large skillet over medium heat. Sauté onions in hot oil 3 minutes, or until tender. Add fish; cook, turning once, until fish is golden brown. Remove and set aside.

In same skillet, sauté spinach 1 minute, or until wilted. Spoon into prepared pan; top with reserved fillets and onions. Sprinkle with salt, nutmeg and pepper. Top with layer of tomatoes, then cheese. Bake 15 minutes, or until heated through and cheese melts. Makes 6 servings.

Per serving: 162 calories; 24 g. protein; 4 g. fat; 23% calories from fat; 51 mg. cholesterol; 7 g. carbohydrates; 331 mg. sodium; 3 g. fiber

Sole with Sweet-Sour Vegetables

1 pound boneless, skinless sole or flounder fillets,
  loosely rolled
1 tablespoon lemon juice
1 tablespoon canola, corn, cottonseed, safflower or
  soybean oil
2 cups julienne-cut carrots (cut 2¼ x ¼-inch)
½ cup thinly sliced onions
2 tablespoons water
2 cups sliced celery
½ cup sliced water chestnuts
1 can (8¼ ounces) pineapple chunks in juice
3 tablespoons cider vinegar
1½ tablespoons brown sugar
1½ tablespoons soy sauce
1½ teaspoons cornstarch

In large skillet over medium-low heat, place fish rolls with enough boiling water to barely cover; add lemon juice. Cover and simmer 8 to 10 minutes, or until fish flakes easily with fork. Keep warm.

Heat oil in another skillet over medium-high heat. Add carrots and onions; cook, stirring constantly, 5 minutes. Reduce heat to medium; add water. Cover and steam 4 minutes. Uncover; add celery and water chestnuts. Cook, stirring constantly, 2 minutes. Add undrained pineapple.

In small bowl, combine remaining ingredients. Add to skillet mixture; cook, stirring, 2 minutes, or until sauce coats vegetables and pineapple. Remove fish rolls from liquid; drain well. Serve fish topped with sweet-sour sauce. Makes 4 servings.

Note: Sauce is also good over broiled or baked fish or poultry.

Per serving: 262 calories; 23 g. protein; 5 g. fat; 17% calories from fat; 54 mg. cholesterol; 31 g. carbohydrates; 588 mg. sodium; 5 g. fiber

Halibut Hawaiian

2 halibut steaks (1 pound each), fresh or thawed frozen
1¾ teaspoons salt
1 cup soft bread cubes
1 cup drained crushed pineapple
1 cup cooked rice
2 tablespoons lemon juice
½ teaspoon curry powder
2 tablespoons butter or margarine, melted

Preheat oven to 350°F. Grease 12 x 8-inch baking dish or pan; set aside. Sprinkle steaks with 1 teaspoon salt. Place 1 steak in prepared dish; set aside. In medium bowl, stir bread cubes, pineapple, rice, lemon juice, remaining ¾ teaspoon salt and curry powder; place over steak. Top with remaining steak. Secure with toothpicks or skewers. Brush top steak with butter or margarine. Bake 30 to 40 minutes, or until fish flakes easily when tested with fork. Makes 6 servings.

Per serving: 271 calories; 32 g. protein; 7 g. fat; 26% calories from fat; 58 mg. cholesterol; 15 g. carbohydrates; 776 mg. sodium; 0 g. fiber

Mediterranean Baked Fish

1   pound boneless, skinless fish fillets (sole, flounder,
        sea perch, turbot)
1   tablespoon corn oil
1   large onion, diced
3   large tomatoes, chopped, or 1 can (16 ounces)
        tomatoes, drained
1   clove garlic, minced
1   cup bottled clam juice
½   cup dry white wine
1   bay leaf
1   tablespoon shredded orange rind
1   teaspoon fennel seeds, crushed
½   teaspoon dried oregano
¼   teaspoon dried thyme
¼   teaspoon dried basil
    Salt and pepper to taste

Preheat oven to 375°F. Grease 11 x 7-inch baking dish; place fish in single layer and set aside. Heat oil in large skillet over medium heat. Sauté onions 3 minutes, or until tender. Add remaining ingredients. Reduce heat to low; simmer, stirring occasionally, in uncovered skillet 30 minutes. Remove bay leaf. Pour sauce over fish. Bake 15 to 20 minutes, or until fish flakes easily with fork. Makes 4 servings.

Per serving: 193 calories; 23 g. protein; 5 g. fat; 24% calories from fat; 54 mg. cholesterol; 8 g. carbohydrates; 231 mg. sodium; 2 g. fiber

Fish in Green Tomato Sauce

2 tablespoons canola, corn, cottonseed, safflower or
   soybean oil
1 large onion, thinly sliced
2 cans Mexican green tomatoes (tomatillos), drained
⅓ cup chopped fresh cilantro
1-2 small hot green chili peppers, seeded
2 pounds boneless fish fillets (red snapper, cod, turbot),
   cut into 2-inch pieces
2 cups thinly sliced zucchini
   Hot cooked rice (optional)
   Nonfat sour cream (optional)

Heat oil in a large skillet over medium heat. Sauté onions 3
minutes, or until tender; remove from pan with slotted spoon
and set aside. In blender or food processor, combine green
tomatoes, cilantro and peppers until of desired consistency.
Place fish in same skillet; top with reserved onions, then green
tomato sauce. Cook over medium heat 5 minutes. Add zucchini;
cook 5 minutes more, or until fish flakes easily when tested
with fork. Serve over rice with dollop of sour cream, if desired.
Makes 8 servings.

Per serving: 147 calories; 20 g. protein; 4 g. fat; 27% calories from fat; 46 mg. cholesterol; 6 g. carbohydrates; 74 mg.
sodium; 2 g. fiber

West African Tuna Casserole

2 cups cooked black-eyed peas
2 tablespoons canola, corn, cottonseed, safflower or
    soybean oil
½ cup finely chopped onions
1 large tomato, chopped
1½-2 teaspoons chopped, seeded hot red pepper
2 cans (6½ ounces) chunk light tuna, drained and flaked
2 tablespoons tomato paste
½ teaspoon salt
½ cup dry bread crumbs
1 tablespoon butter or margarine, melted

Preheat oven to 350°F. Place peas in 9- or 10-inch baking dish. Heat oil in large skillet over medium heat. Sauté onions 3 minutes, or until tender. Spoon over peas with tomatoes and peppers. Cover and bake 15 minutes. Remove from oven; top with tuna, tomato paste and salt. Cover and bake 15 minutes. In small bowl, combine bread crumbs and butter or margarine until well blended; sprinkle over casserole. Uncover and bake 5 minutes more, or until lightly browned. Makes 6 servings.

Per serving: 242 calories; 22 g. protein; 7 g. fat; 28% calories from fat; 36 mg. cholesterol; 21 g. carbohydrates; 459 mg. sodium; 8 g. fiber

Hot Baked Po-Tunas

4   large baking potatoes, baked
2   cans (7 ounces each) solid white tuna, drained and
    flaked
¾   cup light mayonnaise
½   cup plus 2 tablespoons (2½ ounces) shredded
    reduced-fat Cheddar cheese
¼   cup chopped green peppers
¼   cup chopped pimientos
¼   cup chopped green onions
1   egg white, stiffly beaten

Preheat oven to 400°F. Scoop potatoes from skins, leaving
½-inch shell. In medium bowl, mash scooped potatoes; add
tuna, ½ cup mayonnaise, ½ cup cheese, peppers, pimientos and
green onions, stirring until well combined. Spoon back into
shells; bake 10 minutes.

In small bowl with mixer, beat egg white until stiff peaks
form; fold in remaining ¼ cup mayonnaise and 2 tablespoons
cheese. Spoon evenly over stuffed potatoes. Bake 10 minutes
more. Makes 4 servings.

Per serving: 531 calories; 35 g. protein; 18 g. fat; 31% calories from fat; 67 mg. cholesterol; 55 g. carbohydrates; 795 mg.
sodium; 5 g. fiber

Vegetable-Topped Fish Fillets

¼ cup canola, corn, cottonseed, safflower or soybean oil
6 carp, pike or whitefish fillets (4 ounces each)
1 teaspoon salt
¾ teaspoon pepper
2 large tomatoes, diced
1 package (10 ounces) frozen mixed vegetables, thawed
3 medium potatoes (about 1 pound), peeled and diced
2 medium onions, sliced
¼ teaspoon garlic powder

Preheat oven to 425°F. Place oil in 13 x 9-inch baking dish. Place dish in oven until oil is hot. Sprinkle fish with half salt and pepper; place in dish with hot oil. Bake 10 minutes. Add tomatoes, mixed vegetables, potatoes, onions, garlic powder and remaining salt and pepper. Cover. Reduce heat to 350°F. Bake 40 minutes more; remove cover for last 15 minutes. Makes 6 servings.

Per serving: 273 calories; 24 g. protein; 7 g. fat; 24% calories from fat; 65 mg. cholesterol; 27 g. carbohydrates; 463 mg. sodium; 4 g. fiber

Italian Tuna and Peppers for Two

1   can (7 ounces) solid white tuna packed in water
1   large Spanish or other sweet onion, cut in half and
     thinly sliced
2   medium green peppers, thinly sliced
1   cup tomato juice
¼   teaspoon dried oregano

Drain tuna; reserve liquid and flake tuna. In large nonstick skillet over medium heat, combine tuna liquid and remaining ingredients. Cover and simmer 5 minutes. Uncover and cook 5 minutes, or until tomato juice evaporates into thick sauce. Add flaked tuna; toss gently to evenly mix. Heat through. Makes 2 servings.

Per serving: 149 calories; 26 g. protein; 0 g. fat; 5% calories from fat; 46 mg. cholesterol; 9 g. carbohydrates; 737 mg. sodium; 2 g. fiber

DELECTABLE SIDE DISHES

Cucumbers in Dill

 4   medium cucumbers, peeled and thinly sliced
 1   cup boiling water
 ¾   cup nonfat sour cream
 ¼   cup lemon juice
 3   tablespoons minced fresh dill, or 3 teaspoons dried dill
 1½ teaspoons salt
 1   teaspoon sugar
 ⅛   teaspoon pepper

Place cucumbers in medium bowl; pour on boiling water. Let stand 5 minutes; drain. Plunge cucumbers into ice water; drain and place back in bowl. In small bowl, mix remaining ingredients until well blended. Add to cucumbers; toss gently to evenly coat. Cover and chill 30 minutes. Makes 6 servings.

Per serving: 61 calories; 2 g. protein; 0 g. fat; 4% calories from fat; 5 mg. cholesterol; 12 g. carbohydrates; 577 mg. sodium; 2 g. fiber

Marinated Vegetables

1	pound baby carrots, cooked and drained
½	pound green beans, cooked and drained
1	package (10 ounces) frozen asparagus spears, cooked and drained
1	pint cherry tomatoes, cut into halves
1½	cups tomato juice
1	tablespoon lemon juice
1	teaspoon white vinegar
¼	cup thinly sliced green onions
¼	cup finely chopped fresh parsley, or 1 tablespoon dried parsley
1	clove garlic, minced
1	teaspoon salt
	Dash pepper
	Dash hot-pepper sauce

In large, shallow glass baking dish, casserole or plastic container, arrange carrots, green beans, asparagus and tomatoes in separate groups. In medium bowl, stir tomato juice and remaining ingredients until well blended; pour over vegetables. Cover and chill 3 to 4 hours. Makes 8 servings.

Per serving: 48 calories; 3 g. protein; 0 g. fat; 6% calories from fat; 0 mg. cholesterol; 10 g. carbohydrates; 575 mg. sodium; 3 g. fiber

Red Cabbage

2   tablespoons canola, corn, cottonseed, safflower or
     soybean oil
2   small onions, sliced
1   large head red cabbage (about 2 pounds), shredded
2   tablespoons cider vinegar
1   large tart apple, peeled, cored and finely chopped
1   piece (2 ounces) salt pork
½   cup red wine or water
½   cup hot beef broth
1   teaspoon sugar
     Salt to taste

Heat oil in large saucepan or Dutch oven over medium heat. Sauté onions 3 minutes, or until tender. Add cabbage; immediately pour vinegar over cabbage and toss well. Add remaining ingredients, stirring until well blended. Bring to boil. Reduce heat to low; cover and simmer 45 to 60 minutes, or until cabbage is tender-crisp. Makes 8 servings.

Per serving: 120 calories; 3 g. protein; 6 g. fat; 46% calories from fat; 7 mg. cholesterol; 12 g. carbohydrates; 68 mg. sodium; 3 g. fiber

Quick Zucchini—Genoa Style

3 tablespoons canola, corn, cottonseed, safflower or
  soybean oil
4 medium zucchini, cut into thin strips
1 clove garlic, minced
1 tablespoon fresh chopped parsley, or 1 teaspoon
  dried parsley
1 teaspoon dried oregano
1 teaspoon lemon juice
½ teaspoon salt
½ teaspoon pepper

Heat oil in large skillet over medium heat. Sauté zucchini and garlic for 5 minutes, stirring frequently. Add remaining ingredients. Reduce heat to low; cook 5 minutes longer. Makes 4 servings.

Per serving: 107 calories; 1 g. protein; 10 g. fat; 83% calories from fat; 0 mg. cholesterol; 3 g. carbohydrates; 269 mg. sodium; 1 g. fiber

Sautéed Squash and Potatoes

4   tablespoons olive oil
3   large zucchini, sliced
3   large yellow summer squash, sliced
1   large onion, cut into wedges
3   potatoes, peeled if desired and cut into 1-inch cubes
3   medium tomatoes, coarsely chopped (optional)
    Salt to taste
¼   teaspoon Italian seasoning
⅛   teaspoon pepper

Heat oil in large skillet over medium heat. Sauté zucchini, yellow squash, onions and potatoes, stirring frequently, 10 minutes, or until tender. Add tomatoes, if desired. Season with salt, Italian seasoning and pepper. Makes 8 servings.

Per serving: 139 calories; 3 g. protein; 7 g. fat; 44% calories from fat; 0 mg. cholesterol; 17 g. carbohydrates; 9 mg. sodium; 3 g. fiber

Zucchini and Tomato Casserole

4   tablespoons canola, corn, cottonseed, safflower or
       soybean oil
1   small onion, chopped
½   clove garlic, minced
2   medium zucchini, sliced
2   medium tomatoes, peeled and coarsely chopped,
       or 1 cup canned tomatoes, coarsely chopped
½   teaspoon salt
¼   teaspoon dried basil
¼   teaspoon pepper
2   tablespoons grated Parmesan cheese

Heat oil in large ovenproof skillet over medium heat. Sauté onions and garlic 3 minutes, or until tender. Add zucchini. Reduce heat to low; cover and cook 5 minutes, or until tender-crisp. Add tomatoes, salt, basil and pepper. Cook, uncovered, 10 minutes, or until of desired doneness. Preheat broiler. Sprinkle with cheese. Broil until top is lightly browned. Makes 4 servings.

Per serving: 159 calories; 2 g. protein; 14 g. fat; 80% calories from fat; 2 mg. cholesterol; 5 g. carbohydrates; 320 mg. sodium; 2 g. fiber

Spanish Carrots

2   tablespoons butter or margarine
1   small clove garlic, minced
1   pound young carrots (about 7 or 8), cut diagonally
     ¼-inch thick
¼   teaspoon salt
¼   large green pepper, cut into strips
1   tablespoon catsup
     Chili powder to taste

Melt butter or margarine in large skillet over medium heat. Sauté garlic for 1 minute. Add carrots and salt; cook, tightly covered, 10 minutes, shaking pan occasionally. Add peppers, catsup and chili powder; cook 5 minutes more, or until carrots are tender-crisp. Makes 4 servings.

Per serving: 105 calories; 1 g. protein; 6 g. fat; 49% calories from fat; 15 mg. cholesterol; 12 g. carbohydrates; 266 mg. sodium; 3 g. fiber

Zucchini with Dill Sauce

4   cups sliced zucchini
1   teaspoon dried dill
1   package (1.25 ounces) sour cream sauce mix
½   cup cold skim milk
2   teaspoons lemon juice

In medium saucepan over medium heat, cook zucchini and ½ teaspoon dill in ½ cup lightly salted water for 3 minutes, or until tender-crisp; drain well. Return to saucepan; keep warm.

In small bowl, place sour cream sauce mix and milk; with spoon, beat 1 to 1½ minutes, or until well blended. Let stand 10 minutes. Stir in lemon juice and remaining ½ teaspoon dill; pour over zucchini. Cook 3 to 4 minutes, or until heated through. Makes 4 servings.

Per serving: 104 calories; 5 g. protein; 3 g. fat; 25% calories from fat; 12 mg. cholesterol; 13 g. carbohydrates; 146 mg. sodium; 2 g. fiber

Hot Brussels Sprouts in Dilled "Hollandaise" Sauce

1   package (10 ounces) fresh or frozen Brussels sprouts
    Onion salt to taste
    Pepper to taste
½   cup water
2   tablespoons light mayonnaise
¼   teaspoon dried dill

In medium saucepan over medium heat, cook Brussels sprouts, onion salt, pepper and water 7 to 10 minutes, or until sprouts are tender-crisp. With slotted spoon, remove Brussels sprouts to serving bowl; keep warm.

Add mayonnaise and dill to seasoned water, stirring until well blended. Cook, uncovered, until of desired sauce consistency; pour over warm sprouts. Makes 3 servings.

Per serving: 73 calories; 3 g. protein; 3 g. fat; 41% calories from fat; 3 mg. cholesterol; 8 g. carbohydrates; 98 mg. sodium; 4 g. fiber

Zucchini and Cheese Bake

8 ounces low-fat cottage cheese
½ teaspoon dried basil
2 tablespoons canola, corn, cottonseed, safflower or soybean oil
2 medium zucchini, sliced
1 small onion, chopped
2 tablespoons grated Parmesan cheese

Preheat oven to 350°F. Grease 1½-quart casserole; set aside. In food processor or blender, puree cottage cheese and basil until smooth; set aside. Heat oil in large skillet over medium heat. Sauté zucchini and onions 3 minutes, or until crisp-tender; drain. In prepared casserole, place layer of ½ zucchini, then ½ cheese mixture; repeat. Top with Parmesan cheese. Bake 20 to 25 minutes, or until heated through. Makes 4 servings.

Per serving: 90 calories; 2 g. protein; 7 g. fat; 73% calories from fat; 2 mg. cholesterol; 4 g. carbohydrates; 49 mg. sodium; 1 g. fiber

Brown Rice Cheese Strata

1   cup uncooked brown rice
1   cup low-fat cottage cheese
2   tablespoons chopped pimientos
1   egg, beaten
¼   teaspoon salt
2   tablespoons butter or margarine
½   cup sliced celery
½   cup sliced onions
2   cups shredded reduced-fat Cheddar cheese
    Paprika to taste
    Tomato slices or green pepper rings for garnish
    (optional)

Preheat oven to 375°F. Cook rice according to package directions. In large bowl, stir cooked rice, cottage cheese, pimientos, egg and salt until well blended. Melt butter or margarine in small skillet over medium heat. Sauté celery and onions for 3 minutes, or until onions are tender. Stir into rice mixture.

In 2-quart casserole, spoon ½ rice mixture; sprinkle with 1 cup Cheddar cheese. Repeat layers. Cover and bake 25 to 30 minutes, or until heated through. Sprinkle with paprika. Top with tomato slices or pepper rings, if desired. Makes 6 servings.

Per serving: 284 calories; 18 g. protein; 11 g. fat; 36% calories from fat; 74 mg. cholesterol; 28 g. carbohydrates; 538 mg. sodium; 1 g. fiber

Orange Rice

2 tablespoons butter or margarine
½ cup thinly sliced celery
3 tablespoons finely chopped onions
1½ cups water
1 cup orange juice
2 tablespoons shredded orange peel
½ teaspoon salt
Pepper to taste
1 cup uncooked long-grain rice

Melt butter or margarine in medium saucepan over medium heat. Sauté celery and onions 3 minutes, or until tender. Add water, orange juice, orange peel, salt and pepper. Bring to boil. Add rice. Reduce heat to low; cover and cook 20 minutes, or until rice is tender. Makes 6 servings.

Per serving: 170 calories; 2 g. protein; 4 g. fat; 22% calories from fat; 20 mg. cholesterol; 30 g. carbohydrates; 222 mg. sodium; 1 g. fiber

Arroz Verde

1   small bunch parsley
3   sprigs cilantro
2   large romaine lettuce leaves, torn into pieces
2   canned green chilies
¼   small onion, chopped
½   cup water
⅓   cup canola, corn, cottonseed, safflower or soybean oil
1½   cups uncooked long-grain rice
3   cups defatted chicken broth or bouillon

In blender or food processor, puree parsley, cilantro, lettuce, chilies, onions and water until smooth; set aside.

Heat oil in large skillet over medium heat. Add rice and cook, stirring, until golden. Drain off excess oil. Add pureed parsley mixture; cook, stirring, until rice is almost dry. Add broth or bouillon; cook, uncovered, 15 minutes, or until all liquid is absorbed. Cover and let stand 5 minutes, or until ready to serve. Makes 8 servings.

Per serving: 220 calories; 4 g. protein; 8 g. fat; 37% calories from fat; 0 mg. cholesterol; 29 g. carbohydrates; 298 mg. sodium; 1 g. fiber

Spanish Rice

2   tablespoons canola, corn, cottonseed, safflower or
    soybean oil
2   tablespoons diced onions
2   tablespoons diced green peppers
1   can (16 ounces) tomatoes
1   can (8 ounces) tomato sauce
2   beef bouillon cubes
2   teaspoons chili powder
    Salt and pepper to taste
    Worcestershire sauce to taste
1   cup uncooked long-grain rice

Heat oil in large skillet over medium heat. Sauté onions and peppers 5 minutes, or until slightly brown. Add tomatoes, tomato sauce, bouillon, chili powder, salt, pepper and Worcestershire sauce. Bring to boil. Add rice. Reduce heat to low; cover and simmer, stirring occasionally, 20 to 30 minutes, or until rice is done. Makes 6 servings.

Per serving: 186 calories; 3 g. protein; 5 g. fat; 25% calories from fat; 0 mg. cholesterol; 31 g. carbohydrates; 694 mg. sodium; 2 g. fiber

Parsley Rice

1   cup uncooked rice
2   cups water
2   chicken bouillon cubes
1   teaspoon salt
2   teaspoons butter or margarine
⅓   cup minced green peppers
¼   cup sliced green onions
¼   cup chopped slivered almonds
½   cup chopped parsley

In medium saucepan over medium heat, cook rice in water, bouillon and salt for 15 minutes, or until rice is tender. Melt butter or margarine in small saucepan over medium heat. Sauté peppers, green onions and almonds for 3 minutes. Stir into rice with parsley. Makes 6 servings.

Per serving: 167 calories; 3 g. protein; 4 g. fat; 24% calories from fat; 3 mg. cholesterol; 27 g. carbohydrates; 636 mg. sodium; 2 g. fiber

Curried Rice with Peas

2   cans (13¾ ounces each) ready-to-use chicken broth
1¾ cups uncooked long-grain rice
1   package (10 ounces) frozen peas
2   tablespoons canola, corn, cottonseed, safflower or
      soybean oil
1   tablespoon curry powder
2   teaspoons salt

Preheat oven to 350°F. Grease 3-quart casserole. Place all ingredients in casserole; stir until well mixed. Cover and bake 1 hour, or until rice is tender. Fluff mixture with fork before serving. Makes 10 servings.

Per serving: 203 calories; 5 g. protein; 6 g. fat; 28% calories from fat; 0 mg. cholesterol; 30 g. carbohydrates; 705 mg. sodium; 2 g. fiber

Black-Eyed Peas Supreme

2 cans (16 ounces each) black-eyed peas, drained
1 onion, thinly sliced into rings
¼ cup olive oil
¼ cup wine vinegar
1 clove garlic, minced
1 tablespoon Worcestershire sauce
1 teaspoon salt
   Pepper to taste

Place peas and onions in medium bowl; set aside. In small saucepan over high heat, bring to boil remaining ingredients; pour immediately over peas and onions. Cover and chill several hours or overnight. Makes 8 servings.

Per serving: 134 calories; 4 g. protein; 7 g. fat; 48% calories from fat; 0 mg. cholesterol; 13 g. carbohydrates; 551 mg. sodium; 6 g. fiber

Tomato Sauced Green Beans and Potatoes

1   tablespoon canola oil
1   clove garlic, minced
1   package (10 ounces) frozen cut green beans, or
    1 can (16 ounces) cut green beans, drained
2   medium potatoes, cut into 1-inch cubes
1   can (8 ounces) tomato sauce
    Salt and pepper to taste
    French or Italian bread (optional)

Heat oil in large skillet over medium heat. Sauté garlic for 3 minutes, or until brown. Add green beans, potatoes, tomato sauce, salt and pepper. Bring to boil. Reduce heat to low; cover and simmer 20 to 25 minutes, or until vegetables are fork-tender. Serve with bread, if desired. Makes 4 servings.

Per serving: 124 calories; 2 g. protein; 3 g. fat; 25% calories from fat; 0 mg. cholesterol; 21 g. carbohydrates; 355 mg. sodium; 4 g. fiber

Make-Believe "Sweet Potatoes"

2   packages (10 ounces each) frozen sliced yellow squash
    Sugar or artificial sweetener to taste
½   teaspoon ground cinnamon
½   teaspoon ground ginger
⅛   teaspoon salt
1   tablespoon butter or margarine (optional)

In large saucepan over medium heat, bring to boil squash and ½ cup water; cook 10 minutes, or until tender. Drain. In serving bowl, place hot cooked squash, enough sugar or artificial sweetener to sweeten, cinnamon, ginger and salt; toss gently to evenly coat. If desired, top with butter or margarine. Makes 6 servings.

Per serving: 20 calories; 1 g. protein; 0 g. fat; 8% calories from fat; 0 mg. cholesterol; 4 g. carbohydrates; 44 mg. sodium; 1 g. fiber

Oven French Fries

1   tablespoon oil
1   tablespoon water
3   medium potatoes, peeled and cut into thin strips

Preheat oven to 475°F. In medium bowl, mix oil and water; add potatoes, turning until well coated. On large baking sheet lined with foil, place potatoes in single layer. Bake 25 to 30 minutes, or until potatoes are cooked. Makes 4 servings.

Per serving: 154 calories; 2 g. protein; 3 g. fat; 20% calories from fat; 0 mg. cholesterol; 28 g. carbohydrates; 8 mg. sodium; 2 g. fiber

Broccoli with Tart Sauce

1 head broccoli or broccoflower (about 1 pound),
   separated into florets
2 tablespoons butter or margarine, melted
1½ teaspoons prepared white horseradish
1½ teaspoons sugar
½ teaspoon salt
½ teaspoon paprika

In large saucepan over medium heat, bring to boil broccoli or broccoflower and ½ cup water. Reduce heat to medium; cook 10 minutes, or until tender. Drain. In serving bowl, stir remaining ingredients until well blended. Add broccoli or broccoflower; toss gently to evenly coat. Makes 4 servings.

Per serving: 91 calories; 3 g. protein; 6 g. fat; 54% calories from fat; 15 mg. cholesterol; 8 g. carbohydrates; 329 mg. sodium; 3 g. fiber

Italian-Style Broccoli Pasta

1   cup uncooked elbow macaroni or other small pasta
2   cups coarsely chopped cooked broccoli or broccoflower
2   tablespoons olive oil
1   small clove garlic, minced
    Salt to taste

Cook macaroni or other pasta according to package directions; drain and place into large serving bowl. Immediately toss with remaining ingredients. Serve immediately. Makes 4 servings.

Per serving: 86 calories; 2 g. protein; 6 g. fat; 66% calories from fat; 0 mg. cholesterol; 5 g. carbohydrates; 22 mg. sodium; 2 g. fiber

Stuffed Celery

½   cup low-fat cottage cheese
⅓   cup chopped sweet gherkins (about 2)
1   tablespoon chopped celery leaves
¼   teaspoon Worcestershire sauce
¼   teaspoon salt
6   ribs celery, cut into 8-inch pieces

In small bowl, stir cottage cheese, gherkins, celery leaves, Worcestershire sauce and salt until well mixed. Spread cheese mixture evenly on celery pieces. Makes 6 servings.

Per serving: 36 calories; 2 g. protein; 0 g. fat; 9% calories from fat; 2 mg. cholesterol; 6 g. carbohydrates; 277 mg. sodium; 0 g. fiber

Beans and Sprouts

1 pound green beans, trimmed and cut diagonally
   into ½-inch pieces
¼ cup boiling water
2 tablespoons canola, corn, cottonseed, safflower or
   soybean oil
2 tablespoons sesame oil
1 pound fresh mung-bean sprouts
½ cup loosely packed thinly sliced Spanish or other
   sweet onions
2 tablespoons minced fresh ginger
1 clove garlic, minced
3 tablespoons soy sauce mixed with 2 teaspoons sugar

In wok or large heavy skillet over high heat, bring to boil green beans, water and oils. Reduce heat; partially cover and simmer 5 to 8 minutes, or until beans are tender-crisp and water has evaporated. Add bean sprouts, onions, ginger, garlic and soy sauce mixture; cook, stirring constantly, 1 minute, or until onions are tender-crisp. Makes 8 servings.

Per serving: 105 calories; 3 g. protein; 7 g. fat; 55% calories from fat; 0 mg. cholesterol; 9 g. carbohydrates; 392 mg. sodium; 3 g. fiber

Tomatoes Stuffed with Spinach

5   medium tomatoes
½   teaspoon salt
2   packages (10 ounces each) frozen chopped spinach
2   tablespoons butter or margarine
1   small onion, grated
½   cup nonfat sour cream
¼   cup grated Parmesan cheese
    Pepper to taste
    Dash cayenne pepper to taste
⅓   cup Italian-seasoned dry bread crumbs

Preheat oven to 350°F. Grease baking dish large enough to hold tomatoes; set aside. Cut tops off tomatoes; scoop out pulp, reserving for another use, leaving ½-inch shell. Sprinkle with ¼ teaspoon salt; invert to drain.

Meanwhile, cook spinach according to package directions. Drain; cool, then squeeze dry. Melt 1 tablespoon butter or margarine in medium skillet over medium heat. Sauté onions 3 minutes, or until tender. Stir in spinach, sour cream, cheese, remaining ¼ teaspoon salt and peppers. Spoon into tomato shells. Place in prepared pan. Sprinkle top with bread crumbs; dot with remaining tablespoon butter or margarine. Bake 20 to 25 minutes, or until heated through. Makes 5 servings.

Per serving: 137 calories; 8 g. protein; 3 g. fat; 20% calories from fat; 9 mg. cholesterol; 21 g. carbohydrates; 379 mg. sodium; 5 g. fiber

Spiced Garbanzo Beans

3   tablespoons canola, corn, cottonseed, safflower or
       soybean oil
1   medium onion, finely chopped
1   clove garlic, finely chopped
1   tomato, peeled and chopped
2   jalapeño peppers, seeded and chopped
2   teaspoons chili powder
¼   teaspoon dried oregano
1   can (15 to 19 ounces) garbanzo beans (chickpeas),
       drained
       Salt to taste

Heat oil in large skillet over medium heat. Cook onions and garlic for 3 minutes. Add tomatoes, peppers, chili powder and oregano. Cook over low heat, stirring frequently, 10 minutes, or until most liquid has evaporated. Add garbanzo beans and salt; cover and simmer 20 minutes more. Makes 6 servings.

Per serving: 172 calories; 5 g. protein; 8 g. fat; 43% calories from fat; 0 mg. cholesterol; 19 g. carbohydrates; 7 mg. sodium; 4 g. fiber

Hungarian Asparagus

1   pound fresh trimmed asparagus, cooked, or 2 packages
     (10 ounces each) frozen asparagus spears, cooked
¼   cup nonfat sour cream
1   cup buttered bread crumbs*

Preheat oven to 350°F. Grease 11 x 7-inch baking dish or
2½-quart shallow casserole; arrange asparagus in single layer.
Cover with sour cream, then bread crumbs. Bake about 15
minutes, or until bread crumbs are golden brown. Serves 6.

To make buttered crumbs: Heat 3 tablespoons butter, margarine or oil until hot in small saucepan over medium heat.
Add 1 cup bread crumbs. Cook, stirring, until crumbs are lightly browned.

Per serving: 143 calories; 5 g. protein; 3 g. fat; 41% calories
from fat; 18 mg. cholesterol; 16 g. carbohydrates; 186 mg.
sodium; 1 g. fiber

Stuffed Mushrooms

1½   pounds large fresh mushrooms (about 24)
2   tablespoons butter or margarine
1   large onion, finely chopped
½   cup Italian-seasoned dry bread crumbs

Preheat oven to 350°F. Remove mushroom stems; finely chop and set aside. Melt butter or margarine in small saucepan over medium heat. Sauté onions 3 minutes, or until tender. Add chopped mushrooms. Cook 3 minutes, or until tender. Add bread crumbs, stirring until well combined. On large baking or jelly-roll pan, place mushroom caps top-side down; fill with bread crumb mixture. Add enough water to cover bottom of pan. Bake 20 minutes, or until mushrooms are tender. Makes 6 servings.

Per serving: 93 calories; 3 g. protein; 4 g. fat; 41% calories from fat; 10 mg. cholesterol; 11 g. carbohydrates; 74 mg. sodium; 3 g. fiber

Stewed Okra and Tomatoes

2   tablespoons canola, corn, cottonseed, safflower or
     soybean oil
1   small onion, chopped
1   package (10 ounces) frozen okra
1   can (16 ounces) tomatoes, undrained
½   teaspoon salt
¼   teaspoon pepper

Heat oil in large saucepan over medium heat. Sauté onions 5 minutes, or until lightly browned. Add remaining ingredients. Cook, stirring occasionally, 10 to 15 minutes, or until okra is tender. Makes 6 servings.

Per serving: 76 calories; 2 g. protein; 5 g. fat; 53% calories from fat; 0 mg. cholesterol; 8 g. carbohydrates; 302 mg. sodium; 2 g. fiber

Italian Peppers

2   cups chopped red and/or green peppers
1   can (8 ounces) tomatoes, broken up
3   tablespoons chopped onions
    Pinch dried oregano or pizza herbs
    Grated Parmesan or Romano cheese (optional)

In large saucepan over medium heat, combine peppers, tomatoes, onions and oregano or herbs; cover and simmer 5 minutes. Uncover; cook until thickened to desired sauce consistency. Top with cheese, if desired. Makes 4 servings.

Note: To bake in oven, if desired: Preheat oven to 425°F. In 1½-quart casserole, combine all ingredients except cheese. Cover and bake 20 to 25 minutes. Top with cheese.

Per serving: 25 calories; 1 g. protein; 0 g. fat; 12% calories from fat; 0 mg. cholesterol; 5 g. carbohydrates; 94 mg. sodium; 1 g. fiber

Green Bean–Mushroom Casserole

2 packages (10 ounces each) frozen cut green beans
¼ cup finely chopped onions
1 teaspoon salt
1 can (10½ ounces) condensed cream of
    mushroom soup
1 can (4 ounces) mushroom stems and pieces,
    drained and chopped
½ cup canned French-fried onion rings

Preheat oven to 350°F. Grease 1½-quart casserole; set aside. In large saucepan over medium heat, bring to boil ¼ cup water, green beans and onions. Cook 12 minutes, or until tender. Drain; return to saucepan. Stir in undiluted soup and mushrooms; pour into prepared casserole. Top with onion rings. Cover and bake 30 minutes, or until mixture is heated through. Uncover last 5 minutes to brown top. Makes 6 servings.

Per serving: 123 calories; 3 g. protein; 6 g. fat; 47% calories from fat; 1 mg. cholesterol; 13 g. carbohydrates; 1051 mg. sodium; 4 g. fiber

Tossed Rice Bowl

1	clove garlic, cut in half
1	can (16 ounces) bean sprouts, drained and rinsed
1	cup thinly sliced radishes
1	cup diced unpeeled cucumbers
1	cup thinly sliced celery
1	cup chopped watercress or lettuce
2	small Spanish or other sweet onions, chopped
¼	cup chopped green peppers
1½	cups cold cooked rice
1	cup light mayonnaise
	Soy sauce to taste (optional)

Rub garlic on sides of large salad bowl. Layer vegetables and rice in order given. Top with mayonnaise. Just before serving, toss gently to blend well. Serve with soy sauce, if desired. Makes 6 servings.

Per serving: 206 calories; 2 g. protein; 13 g. fat; 60% calories from fat; 13 mg. cholesterol; 18 g. carbohydrates; 342 mg. sodium; 3 g. fiber

Mexican-Style Beans

1   package (16 ounces) pinto beans, rinsed and
    picked over
2   cups chopped tomatoes
1   medium onion, diced
1   can or jar (12 ounces) prepared taco sauce
1   can (4 ounces) green chilies, chopped
2   cloves garlic, minced
1½ teaspoons salt
½   teaspoon ground cumin
½   teaspoon pepper

In large saucepot or Dutch oven, place beans and enough water to cover by 2 inches. Let stand overnight, or boil 2 minutes, then let stand 1 hour. Stir in remaining ingredients. Bring to boil. Reduce heat to low; cover and simmer 1½ to 3 hours, or until beans are tender, adding boiling water if needed. Makes 12 servings.

Per serving: 128 calories; 7 g. protein; 0 g. fat; 4% calories from fat; 0 mg. cholesterol; 24 g. carbohydrates; 430 mg. sodium; 9 g. fiber

Tomatoes Provençales

1½ cups soft bread crumbs
¾ cup finely minced onions
¾ cup chopped parsley
2 tablespoons olive oil
3 cloves garlic, minced
1 teaspoon salt
¾ teaspoon dried thyme, crumbled
⅛ teaspoon pepper
2 pints cherry tomatoes

Preheat oven to 425°F. Grease shallow baking dish large enough to hold tomatoes in single layer; set aside. In medium bowl, combine bread crumbs, onions, parsley, oil, garlic, salt, thyme and pepper until well blended. Place tomatoes in prepared pan. Sprinkle bread crumb mixture over tomatoes; bake for 8 to 10 minutes, or until tomatoes are fork-tender. Makes 6 servings.

Per serving: 123 calories; 2 g. protein; 7 g. fat; 53% calories from fat; 0 mg. cholesterol; 12 g. carbohydrates; 426 mg. sodium; 3 g. fiber

Vegetable Medley

¼ cup butter or margarine, melted
½ cup cornflake crumbs
¼ cup grated Parmesan cheese
1 cup French-cut green beans
1 cup cauliflower florets, cooked
1 cup sliced carrots, cooked
2 teaspoons instant minced onions
1 cup (4 ounces) shredded reduced-fat Cheddar cheese
1 can (10½ ounces) condensed cream of
     mushroom soup
1 cup sliced potatoes, cooked

Preheat oven to 350°F. Grease 11 x 7-inch (1½-quart) baking dish; set aside. In small bowl, combine butter or margarine, cornflake crumbs and Parmesan cheese until well mixed; set aside. In prepared baking dish, place green beans, cauliflower, carrots and onions. Add Cheddar cheese and soup; stir until well mixed. Arrange potatoes in layer over vegetable mixture. Evenly top with crumb mixture. Bake 30 minutes, or until thoroughly heated. Makes 8 servings.

Per serving: 186 calories; 7 g. protein; 12 g. fat; 60% calories from fat; 23 mg. cholesterol; 11 g. carbohydrates; 739 mg. sodium; 2 g. fiber

Braised Leeks

3   bunches leeks, cut in half lengthwise and well rinsed
2   tablespoons butter or margarine
1   medium Bermuda onion, thinly sliced
2   cups beef broth or bouillon
2   whole cloves
1   bay leaf
½   teaspoon salt
⅛   teaspoon pepper

Cut off tops of leeks within 1½ inches of white part; save tops for another use. Melt butter or margarine in large skillet over medium heat. Sauté onions 5 minutes, or until lightly browned. Add leeks and remaining ingredients. Partially cover and simmer 30 minutes, or until leeks are tender and broth has almost evaporated. Remove cloves and bay leaf. Makes 6 servings.

Per serving: 136 calories; 2 g. protein; 4 g. fat; 27% calories from fat; 10 mg. cholesterol; 23 g. carbohydrates; 274 mg. sodium; 4 g. fiber

Orange-Buttered Acorn Squash

2 medium acorn squash, cut in half and seeded
½ teaspoon salt
2 tablespoons firmly packed brown sugar
2 tablespoons butter or margarine
¼ cup orange juice

Preheat oven to 350°F. In 13 x 9-inch baking dish, place squash cut-side down. Bake 40 minutes; turn cut-side up. Sprinkle with salt; into each cavity, place ½ tablespoon brown sugar, ½ tablespoon butter or margarine and 1 tablespoon orange juice. Return to oven; bake 15 to 20 minutes more, or until squash is fork-tender. Makes 4 servings.

Per serving: 152 calories, 1 g. protein; 4 g. fat; 33% calories from fat; 15 mg. cholesterol; 26 g. carbohydrates; 324 mg. sodium; 3 g. fiber

DELICIOUS DESSERTS

Cranberry Ice

1   can (8 ounces) jellied cranberry sauce
1-2   drops red food coloring
½   cup lemon-lime carbonated beverage

In small bowl with mixer, beat cranberry sauce and food coloring until smooth. Slowly beat in lemon-lime beverage. Pour into small refrigerator tray. Cover and freeze until firm. In chilled small mixer bowl, break up cranberry mixture into chunks; beat until fluffy. Return to tray. Cover and refreeze. To serve, scoop into dessert glasses. Makes 2 servings.

Per serving: 196 calories; 0 g. protein; 0 g. fat; 1% calories from fat; 0 mg. cholesterol; 50 g. carbohydrates; 39 mg. sodium; 2 g. fiber

Three-Fruit Salad

1 apple (Red Delicious, Gala), cored, unpeeled and
   cut into small pieces
1 banana, peeled and sliced
¼ cup pineapple chunks, drained
¼ cup nonfat plain yogurt
1 tablespoon pineapple juice
1 teaspoon sugar
⅛ teaspoon nutmeg
   Lettuce for garnish (optional)

In small bowl, mix apples, bananas and pineapple. For dressing, in another small bowl, mix yogurt, pineapple juice, sugar and nutmeg until well blended. Pour over fruit; toss gently to coat. Serve on bed of lettuce, if desired. Makes 4 servings.

Per serving: 76 calories; 1 g. protein; 0 g. fat; 4% calories from fat; 0 mg. cholesterol; 18 g. carbohydrates; 11 mg. sodium; 2 g. fiber

Melon Cooler

1   package (4-serving size) lemon gelatin
1   cup hot water
1   cup cold water
1   tablespoon lemon juice
1½ cups melon balls (cantaloupe, honeydew)
    Additional melon balls and lettuce for garnish (optional)

In medium bowl, stir gelatin and hot water until gelatin is dissolved. Add cold water and lemon juice. Chill until slightly thickened; fold in melon balls. Turn into 1-quart mold or bowl; chill until firm. To serve, unmold onto serving platter. Place melon balls and lettuce around mold, if desired. Makes 6 servings.

Per serving: 68 calories; 1 g. protein; 0 g. fat; 1% calories from fat; 0 mg. cholesterol; 16 g. carbohydrates; 39 mg. sodium; trace g. fiber

Jellied Blueberries and Peaches

1   envelope unflavored gelatin
½   cup cold water
1   cup boiling water
⅓   cup sugar
¼   cup fresh lime juice
¼   teaspoon grated lime peel
1   cup fresh blueberries
1   cup ¼-inch cubes peeled peaches

In medium bowl, sprinkle gelatin over cold water; let stand 5 minutes, or until softened. Stir in boiling water, sugar, lime juice and lime peel until gelatin and sugar dissolve. Chill until slightly thickened. In small bowl, gently stir blueberries and peaches; fold into gelatin mixture. Spoon into 6 individual ½-cup dessert dishes or glasses. Chill until firm. Makes 6 servings.

Per serving: 75 calories; 1 g. protein; 0 g. fat; 2% calories from fat; 0 mg. cholesterol; 18 g. carbohydrates; 2 mg. sodium; 1 g. fiber

Red, White and Blue Mold

2   packages (4-serving size) strawberry gelatin
3   cups boiling water
1   package (10 ounces) frozen strawberries in syrup, thawed
2   packages (4-serving size) lemon gelatin
1   can (15¼ ounces) crushed pineapple in juice
4   cups nonfat sour cream
2   packages (4-serving size) black cherry gelatin
3   cups fresh or canned blueberries

For red layer: In medium bowl, stir strawberry gelatin and 1 cup boiling water until gelatin is dissolved. In 4-cup measure, place strawberries and syrup; add enough water to make 4 cups. Stir into dissolved gelatin. Pour into 16-cup mold or bowl. Chill until firm, about 4 hours.

For white layer: In medium bowl, stir lemon gelatin and 1 cup boiling water until gelatin is dissolved. In 4-cup measure, place pineapple and juice; add enough water to make 3 cups. Stir into dissolved gelatin with 2 cups sour cream. Pour into mold over strawberry layer. Chill until firm, about 4 hours.

For blue layer: In medium bowl, stir black cherry gelatin and 1 cup boiling water until gelatin is dissolved. In 4-cup measure, place blueberries; add enough water to make 3 cups. Stir into dissolved gelatin with remaining 2 cups sour cream. Pour into mold over pineapple layer. Chill until firm, about 4 hours. To serve, unmold onto serving platter. Makes 24 servings.

Per serving: 154 calories; 3 g. protein; 0 g. fat; 1% calories from fat; 6 mg. cholesterol; 34 g. carbohydrates; 109 mg. sodium; 1 g. fiber

Sparkling Dainties

1   package (4-serving size) sugar-free imitation flavor
      gelatin dessert
½   cup boiling water
2   tablespoons nonfat dry milk powder

In 8-inch baking dish or pan, stir gelatin and boiling water until gelatin is dissolved. Chill until firm. Cut into 1-inch squares; roll in milk powder to coat. Makes 64 dainties.

Per serving: 0 calories; 0 g. protein; 0 g. fat; 0% calories from fat; 0 mg. cholesterol; 0 g. carbohydrates; 0 mg. sodium; 0 g. fiber

Cantaloupe Frappé

1   medium ripe cantaloupe, peeled, seeded and cubed
¼   cup dry sherry (optional)
2   tablespoons honey
2   tablespoons lemon juice
      Fresh mint leaves for garnish (optional)

In blender or food processor, puree cantaloupe cubes in batches until smooth. In medium bowl, stir cantaloupe puree, sherry, if desired, honey and lemon juice. Chill well and serve soft or freeze to thicker frappé stage. To serve, spoon into dessert dishes or glasses. Top with mint sprigs, if desired. Makes 8 servings.

Per serving: 40 calories; 0 g. protein; 0 g. fat; 4% calories from fat; 0 mg. cholesterol; 10 g. carbohydrates; 6 mg. sodium; trace g. fiber

Raspberry Lime Float

½ cup fresh or frozen unsweetened raspberries
¾ cup prepared lemonade
¼ cup (1 scoop) lime sherbet

In tall glass, place raspberries; pour in lemonade. Top with sherbet. Serve with long spoon. Makes 1 serving.

Note: Other fruit, such as blueberries, banana slices, or strawberries may be substituted.

Per serving: 172 calories; 1 g. protein; 1 g. fat; 7% calories from fat; 3 mg. cholesterol; 41 g. carbohydrates; 23 mg. sodium; 4 g. fiber

Ambrosia

1 can (8 ounces) mandarin orange segments, drained
1 can (8 ounces) pineapple tidbits, drained
1½ cups (about 8 ounces) green seedless grapes
2¼ cups (about 8 ounces) miniature marshmallows
1 container (8 ounces) nonfat sour cream
1⅓ cups shredded or flaked coconut
Maraschino cherries for garnish (optional)

Place oranges, pineapple, grapes, marshmallows, sour cream and coconut in large serving bowl; toss gently to coat. Garnish with cherries, if desired. Chill at least 4 hours. Makes 6 servings.

Per serving: 231 calories; 2 g. protein; 5 g. fat; 18% calories from fat; 4 mg. cholesterol; 46 g. carbohydrates; 99 mg. sodium; 3 g. fiber

Upside-Down Cake

½   cup firmly packed brown sugar
1   can (8 ounces) pineapple slices, drained
4   eggs, at room temperature, separated
1   cup sugar
1   cup all-purpose flour
1   teaspoon vanilla extract

Preheat oven to 350°F. Grease 9 x 9-inch or 9-inch round baking pan. Evenly sprinkle with brown sugar; top with pineapple slices and set aside.

In small bowl with mixer, beat egg whites, gradually adding ½ cup sugar until stiff peaks form; set aside.

In large bowl with mixer, beat egg yolks with remaining ½ cup sugar until thick and lemony-looking. Stir in flour until well blended. Fold in egg whites and vanilla until well blended. Spoon into prepared pan. Bake 30 minutes, or until toothpick inserted into center comes out clean. Immediately invert onto serving platter. Makes 8 servings.

Note: If desired, fresh sliced apples or canned or fresh sliced peaches can be substituted for the pineapple.

Per serving: 259 calories; 4 g. protein; 3 g. fat; 10% calories from fat; 137 mg. cholesterol; 54 g. carbohydrates; 41 mg. sodium; trace g. fiber

Carrot Kugel

2   eggs, at room temperature, separated
1   cup cooked or canned diced carrots
⅔   cup sifted cake flour
4   tablespoons sugar
2   tablespoons orange juice
½   teaspoon cinnamon
½   teaspoon salt

Preheat oven to 350°F. Spray 11 x 7-inch baking pan with nonstick cooking spray; set aside. In blender or food processor, place egg yolks and remaining ingredients; blend until smooth. In small bowl with mixer, beat egg whites until stiff peaks form. Fold into carrot mixture. Spoon into prepared pan. Bake 50 to 60 minutes, or until cake pulls away from sides of pan. Cut into squares. Makes 8 servings.

Per serving: 80 calories; 2 g. protein; 1 g. fat; 17% calories from fat; 68 mg. cholesterol; 14 g. carbohydrates; 86 mg. sodium; trace g. fiber

Fresh Harvest Pie

3   large apples peeled, cored and sliced (3 cups)
2   large pears peeled, cored and sliced (2 cups)
1½ cups seedless grapes
½   cup sugar
2   tablespoons all-purpose flour
1   tablespoon lemon juice
½   teaspoon grated lemon peel
½   teaspoon ground cinnamon
¼   teaspoon ground nutmeg
    Pastry for 2-crust pie

Preheat oven to 350°F. In large bowl, place apples, pears, grapes, sugar, flour, lemon juice, lemon peel, cinnamon and nutmeg; mix well.

Divide pastry in half. On lightly floured surface, roll out half of pastry into 12-inch circle. Fit pastry into 9-inch pie plate; trim, leaving 1-inch overhang. Spoon in fruit mixture. Roll remaining pastry into 10-inch circle. Cut pastry into ½-inch strips; weave strips over fruit to form lattice top. Press strips onto bottom crust. Fold crust over strips, forming rim, then flute. Bake for 50 to 60 minutes, or until fruit is tender. Makes 8 servings.

Per serving: 377 calories; 3 g. protein; 14 g. fat; 33% calories from fat; 0 mg. cholesterol; 49 g. carbohydrates; 277 mg. sodium; 3 g. fiber

Pumpkin Pie

⅔ cup sugar
½ teaspoon ground cinnamon
½ teaspoon ground ginger
½ teaspoon ground nutmeg
⅛ teaspoon salt
  Pinch ground cloves
1½ cups canned pumpkin
1½ cups evaporated skim milk
3 egg whites, slightly beaten
1 teaspoon vanilla extract
½ teaspoon grated orange peel
1 unbaked 9-inch pie crust
  Lite nondairy whipped topping for garnish (optional)

Preheat oven to 450°F. In small bowl, mix sugar, cinnamon, ginger, nutmeg, salt and cloves. In large bowl with mixer, beat pumpkin, milk, egg whites, vanilla and orange peel until smooth. Beat in sugar mixture. Pour into pie crust. Bake 10 minutes. Reduce heat to 325°F; bake 45 minutes more, or until knife inserted into center comes out clean. Serve in wedges topped with whipped topping, if desired. Makes 8 servings.

Per serving: 229 calories; 6 g. protein; 7 g. fat; 30% calories from fat; 2 mg. cholesterol; 34 g. carbohydrates; 246 mg. sodium; 1 g. fiber

Bean Bars

1   cup whole-wheat pastry flour
⅓   cup nonfat dry milk powder
½   cup firmly packed brown sugar
1   teaspoon baking soda
1   teaspoon ground cinnamon
½   teaspoon ground nutmeg
½   teaspoon ground cloves
½   teaspoon salt
2   cups cooked or drained canned green beans
1   egg
½   cup canola, cottonseed, safflower or soybean oil
½   cup unsweetened applesauce
¾   cup chopped walnuts
½   cup currants
2   tablespoons confectioners' sugar

Preheat oven to 350°F. Grease 11 x 7-inch baking pan. In large bowl, place flour, milk powder, sugar, baking soda, cinnamon, nutmeg, cloves and salt. In blender or food processor, place green beans, egg, oil and applesauce; process until smooth. Add to flour mixture, stirring until well blended. Stir in walnuts and currants. Pour into prepared pan. Bake 25 to 30 minutes, or until pick inserted into center comes out clean. Sprinkle with confectioners' sugar while warm. Cut into bars. Makes 24 bars.

Per bar: 120 calories; 2 g. protein; 7 g. fat; 52% calories from fat; 11 mg. cholesterol; 13 g. carbohydrates; 90 mg. sodium; 1 g. fiber

Carrot-Date Bars

1   cup whole-wheat pastry flour
1   teaspoon baking powder
½   teaspoon salt
    Cholesterol-free, fat-free egg substitute, equivalent to
       2 eggs
½   cup honey
1   teaspoon vanilla extract
1   cup chopped dates
1   cup shredded carrots
½   cup chopped walnuts

Preheat oven to 350°F. Grease 8 x 8-inch baking pan. In large bowl, mix flour, baking powder and salt. In small bowl, beat egg substitute, honey and vanilla until creamy. Add to flour mixture, stirring until well blended. Stir in dates, carrots and walnuts. Spoon into prepared baking pan; spread evenly. Bake 30 minutes. Cool completely on wire rack; cut into bars. Makes 16 bars.

Per bar: 125 calories; 2 g. protein; 3 g. fat; 22% calories from fat; 34 mg. cholesterol; 23 g. carbohydrates; 99 mg. sodium; 2 g. fiber

Broiled Fruit Cups

6   medium oranges
2   apples, cored, unpeeled and coarsely chopped
1   cup seedless grapes
6   tablespoons sugar

Preheat broiler. With sharp knife, slice tops off oranges. Remove insides of oranges, keeping sections intact. Cut design in edge of shell with kitchen shears, if desired. If necessary, slice small amount off bottom of orange to keep in upright position.

In small bowl, mix orange sections, apples and grapes. Sprinkle with sugar. Fill orange shells with sweetened fruit mixture. Place on broiler pan; broil 6 inches from heat source, or until warm through. Makes 6 servings.

Per serving: 154 calories; 1 g. protein; 0 g. fat; 3% calories from fat; 0 mg. cholesterol; 39 g. carbohydrates; 1 mg. sodium; 4 g. fiber

No-Bake Bran Fruit Squares

3 cups bran flakes cereal
1½ cups chopped raisins
1 cup chopped walnuts
¾ cup chopped dried figs
¾ cup chopped dates
¾ cup sweetened condensed milk
1 tablespoon lemon juice
1 tablespoon honey

In large bowl, mix all ingredients until well blended. Press firmly into 9 x 9-inch baking pan; cut into squares. Remove to platter; let stand 2 hours to dry. Store tightly covered. Makes 36 squares.

Per serving: 93 calories; 1 g. protein; 2 g. fat; 25% calories from fat; 2 mg. cholesterol; 17 g. carbohydrates; 40 mg. sodium; 1 g. fiber

Plum Brulee

4   large plums, cut in half and pitted
¾   cup nonfat sour cream
1   tablespoon granulated sugar
1   teaspoon orange liqueur or ¼ teaspoon grated
     orange peel
¼   teaspoon vanilla extract
⅛   teaspoon ground nutmeg
¼   cup firmly packed brown sugar

Preheat broiler. In small broiler-proof baking dish, place plums cut side up. In small bowl, mix sour cream, sugar, orange liqueur or orange peel, vanilla and nutmeg. Spoon over plum halves. Sprinkle with brown sugar. Broil 6 inches from heat source 5 minutes, or until sugar has melted and plums are heated through. Serve warm or chilled. Makes 4 servings.

Per serving: 158 calories; 2 g. protein; 0 g. fat; 3% calories from fat; 7 mg. cholesterol; 35 g. carbohydrates; 66 mg. sodium; 1 g. fiber

Peachy Yogurt Pie

1   envelope unflavored gelatin
¼   cup cold water
2   tablespoons peach brandy or peach nectar
6   tablespoons sugar
½   cup peach or apricot nectar
1   cup nonfat plain yogurt
1   ready-to-fill graham cracker pie crust
3   cups peeled peach or nectarine slices

In small saucepan, sprinkle gelatin over water; let stand 1 minute to soften. Cook over medium-low heat, stirring, until gelatin dissolves. Stir in brandy or nectar and sugar. In small bowl, stir ½ gelatin-brandy mixture with nectar. Chill 10 to 15 minutes, or until slightly thickened; set aside.

In small bowl, stir remaining gelatin-brandy mixture with yogurt; spoon into pie crust. Freeze to set slightly. Remove from freezer; arrange peach or nectarine slices in overlapping concentric circles on top of yogurt filling. Spoon thickened gelatin mixture over fruit to form glaze. Chill until firm and set. Makes 8 servings.

Per serving: 259 calories; 4 g. protein; 11 g. fat; 37% calories from fat; 0 mg. cholesterol; 37 g. carbohydrates; 262 mg. sodium; 2 g. fiber

Orange Sherbet

1 cup skim milk
2 tablespoons thawed frozen orange juice concentrate
2 tablespoons sugar
4-5 ice cubes

In blender or food processor, process all ingredients until smooth yet still icy. Pour into 2 dessert dishes; freeze about 1 hour, or until of desired consistency. Makes 2 servings.

Note: If desired, sherbet may be put in tall glasses and sipped. Other frozen fruit juice concentrates may be substituted.

Per serving: 119 calories; 4 g. protein; 0 g. fat; 2% calories from fat; 2 mg. cholesterol; 25 g. carbohydrates; 63 mg. sodium; 0 g. fiber

Pineapple Ice

½ cup water
⅓ cup pineapple juice
1 tablespoon lemon juice
1 egg white, at room temperature

In small freezer tray, stir water, pineapple juice and lemon juice; freeze, stirring often, until almost firm. In chilled small mixer bowl, break up fruit mixture into chunks; beat until fluffy. In another small bowl, beat egg white until stiff; fold into pineapple ice. Serve immediately or refreeze. Makes 1 serving.

Per serving: 60 calories; 3 g. protein; 0 g. fat; 1% calories from fat; 0 mg. cholesterol; 12 g. carbohydrates; 50 mg. sodium; trace g. fiber

Fruited Yogurt Parfait

1 can (16 ounces) sliced peaches, drained
2 containers (8 ounces each) nonfat vanilla yogurt
1 cup quartered seedless grapes
2 medium pears, peeled and sliced
1 can (8 ounces) pineapple chunks, drained
   Lite nondairy whipped topping (optional)
4 maraschino cherries (optional)

Reserve 8 peach slices for garnish. In each of 4 parfait glasses, layer ¼ remaining peaches, some yogurt, ¼ grapes, some yogurt, ¼ pears, some yogurt, ¼ pineapple and remaining yogurt. Top with dollop of whipped topping and cherry, if desired. Garnish each with 2 reserved peach slices. Makes 4 servings.

Per serving: 144 calories; 5 g. protein; 0 g. fat; 4% calories from fat; 1 mg. cholesterol; 32 g. carbohydrates; 62 mg. sodium; 3 g. fiber

Frozen Pineapple Yogurt

2   cups nonfat plain yogurt
1   can (6 ounces) undiluted thawed frozen pineapple
      juice concentrate
2   teaspoons vanilla extract
      Sugar or artificial sweetener to taste (optional)

In small bowl, stir yogurt, juice concentrate and vanilla until well blended. Add sugar or artificial sweetener, if desired. Spoon into shallow metal baking pan; freeze, uncovered, until partially frozen. In large bowl with mixer, beat yogurt mixture until slushy; return to chilled pan. Freeze until firm. To serve, soften in refrigerator 30 to 40 minutes before scooping. Makes 5 servings.

VARIATION

Substitute orange juice concentrate or any other unsweetened fruit juice concentrate for pineapple.

Per serving: 112 calories; 5 g. protein; 0 g. fat; 2% calories from fat; 1 mg. cholesterol; 22 g. carbohydrates; 70 mg. sodium; 0 g. fiber